Ayurveda for Beginners

The Alchemy of Ayurveda, Yoga & Natural Food for Anxiety, Tension, Depression, Stress & More

By

Lakshmi Vemuri

*Copyright © 2020 – **Streets of Dream Press***

All Rights Reserved.

Published by:

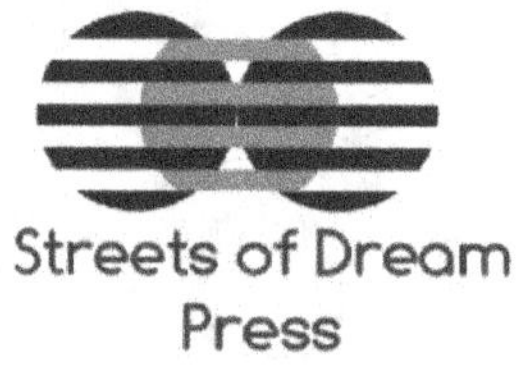

Streets of Dream Press

Cover & Interior designed

By

Jessica Roberts

First Edition

Contents

Ayurveda for Anxiety and Depression: Introduction 12

How Does Ayurveda Work? 18

Techniques Employed in the Practice of Ayurveda 21

Dietary Changes and Mindfulness.................................22

Herbal Medicine..22

Acupressure 23

Massage 24

Meditation 24

Breathing Exercises 25

Panchakarma..26

Sound Therapy 26

Yoga...27

The Fundamentals of Ayurvedic Healing 28

The Three Principle Energies...................................28

Prakruthi 30

Ayurveda as a Complementary Healing System...................30

Ayurveda for Osteoarthritis 31

Ayurveda for Rheumatoid Arthritis..............................32

Ayurveda for Type 2 Diabetes...................................32

Ayurveda for Ulcerative Colitis................................32

Ayurveda for Asthma 33

History, Origin, and Decline of Ayurveda 34

Vedas 36

Texts in Ayurveda 36

Charaka Samhita 37

Sushruta Samhita 38

Ashtanga Hrudhya 38

Sharnagadhara Samhita 39

Bhava Prakasha 40

Madhava Nidanam 40

The Concepts of Ayurveda: Tridhoshic Theory 43

Vata Dosha 44

Pitta Dosha 47

Kapha Dosha 50

Making Sense of the Doshas 53

Vata Types 54

Pitta Types 57

Kapha Types 61

Traits of the Three Doshas 66

Personality Description of Three Doshas 69

Branches of Ayurveda 70

Components of Ayurveda 72

Five Elements Theory or Panchamahabhootha Theory..........73

Ether...73

Air...74

Fire 75

Water 76

Earth...76

Ayurveda and Food...78

Digestion 78

Metabolism 79

Vata Metabolism..80

Pitta Metabolism.......................................80

Kapha Metabolism 81

Wholesome and Unwholesome Foods (Pathya and Apathya)81

Foods That are Wholesome by Nature 82

Foods That are Unwholesome by Nature 82

Best Dietary Habits According to Ayurveda...........83

Steps to Ayurvedic Eating 84

Benefits of Ayurvedic Eating 86

Tips for Good Digestion 87

Foods to Incorporate or Avoid for Different Doshas...........89

Foods Vatas Should Eat 89

Foods Vatas Should Avoid 89

Foods Pittas Should Consume 90

Foods Pittas Should Avoid 90

Foods Kaphas Should Consume 91

Foods Kaphas Should Avoid 91

Eat According to Your Dosha **92**

What is Digestive Fire? **93**

What is Ama? **94**

What is Ojas? **95**

Achieving Balance and Working Out **96**

How Vatas Can Achieve Balance 96

Workouts for Vatas 97

How Pittas Can Achieve Balance 97

Workouts for Pittas 98

How Kaphas Can Achieve Balance 98

Workouts for Kaphas 98

Do's and Don'ts of Ayurveda **99**

Do's of Ayurveda 99

Don'ts of Ayurveda 100

What the Ayurvedic Lifestyle Can Heal ***101***

Anxiety, Stress, and Depression **102**

Depression 104

Stress 105

How to Deal with Anxiety and Depression Using Ayurveda .105

Meditation 105

Lifestyle and Dietary Changes 106

Ayurvedic Herbs 107

Ayurvedic Tools to Deal With Stress, Anxiety, and Depression
...109

Ayurveda & Yoga - a Potent Recipe to Handle Depression and

Anxiety 112

Must-Do Asanas for Complete Well-Being.........................114

Mountain pose: Tadasana..114

Boat pose: Naukasana..115

Warrior pose: Virabhadrasana 116

Powerful pose: Utkatasana..117

Cobra pose: Bhujangasana..118

Mind, Body, and Consciousness 118

Bow pose: Dhanurasana 120

Fish pose: Matsyasana 121

One-legged forward bend: Janu Shirsasana........................122

Bridge pose: Setubandhasana..123

Cat stretch: Marjariasana..124

Two-legged forward bend: Paschimottanasana 125

Downward facing dog: Adhomukha Shwanasana 126

Headstand : Shirshasana 127

Corpse pose: Shavasana 128

Seasonal Yoga Practices **128**

Winter Yoga Practices 129

Summer Yoga Practices 131

Monsoon Yoga Practices 133

Fall Yoga Practices 134

Food and the Mind: Understanding the Mind-Body Connection

.... ***137***

Better Digestion, Better Mood **138**

Ama and Mood **139**

Ayurvedic Tricks for a Better Mind **139**

Write 140

Sip on Herbal Tea 140

Shake Off While You Stand 141

The 6 Tastes of Food **142**

Crafting a Balanced Menu **145**

Compatible and Incompatible Food Combinations............ 146

Eat According to Time and Season 149

Addressing Digestive Imbalances **151**

Ayurvedic Diet Seasonal Guides 154

Autumn/Vata Season Diet....................................155

Summer/Pitta Season Diet....................................158

Spring Season Diet 161

Winter/Kapha Diet 164

Ayurvedic Kitchen Basics....................................166

Chyawanprash 166

Nutritional Facts and Usage 168

Content of Chyawanprash....................................170

Ayurvedic Must-Have Herbs in Your Kitchen 172

Curry Leaves....................................172

Brahmi....................................173

Tulsi/Holy Basil....................................173

Jatamasi/Spikenard 174

Ashwagandha/Indian Ginseng 174

Ayurvedic Must-Have Spices in Your Kitchen....................................174

Cinnamon....................................175

Mustard Seeds 175

Boswellia 176

Asafoetida/Hing 176

Basic Equipment in an Ayurvedic Kitchen....................................177

Ayurvedic Cookware 177

Some Helpful Tips to Follow While Choosing Cooking Vessels

....179

Ayurvedic Pantry Staples 182

Cooking as a Path to Awakening 183

Ayurvedic Recipes to Treat Anxiety and Depression 185

Ayurvedic Teas..186

    CCF Digest Tea...187

    Ginger, Honey, and Lemon Tea...........................188

    Rose Fennel Tea 189

Ayurvedic Tonics...191

    Digestive Lassi 191

    Cucumber Mint Cooler 192

    Golden Milk 194

Ayurvedic Breakfasts 195

    Buckwheat Pancakes...195

    Rice Pudding..197

    Amarnath Chai Porridge....................................199

    Brahmi Pesto...201

Ayurvedic Lunches 203

    Spinach Paneer...203

    Spring Pea Salad...205

    Kitchari 207

Ayurvedic Dinners..**209**

Restorative Shoots & Roots Broth..................................210

Ginger Broccolini 211

Curried Green Beans 213

Ayurvedic Snacks and Sweets **216**

Flatbread Pizza 216

Cauli Tacos 218

Nutty Apple Pie 220

Final Words *224*

Ayurveda for Anxiety and Depression: Introduction

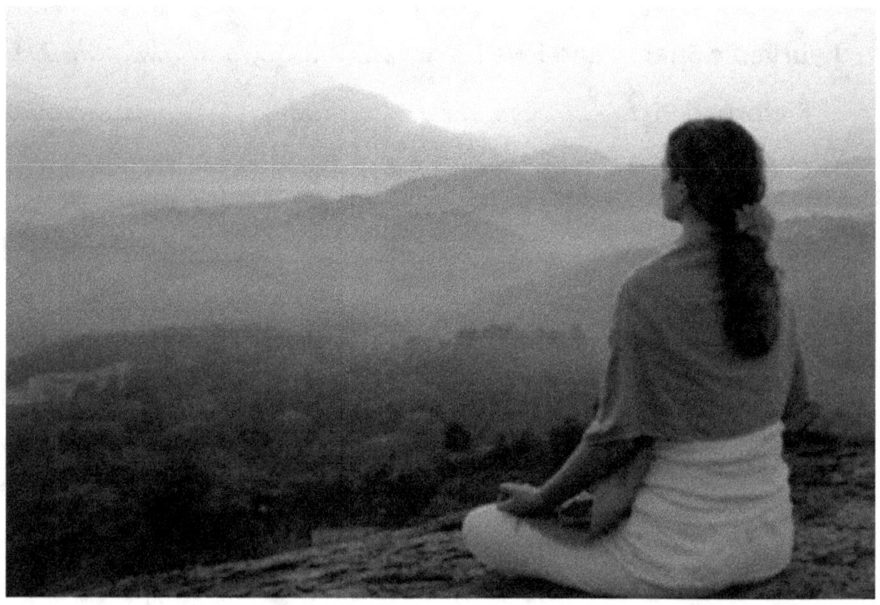

Ayurveda, the oldest health system, has always been a topic of interest for many across the world. However, it hasn't been quite easy to pull up important information about it. Thanks to the internet, we now have access to the world's oldest and probably the first medical system to ever exist.

It all started in the Eastern part of the world. Truth be told, Indians must be given due credit for coming up with such a complex yet practical health system. Oh, I'm talking about the Ancient Indian civilization, which has been in existence for the last few thousand years. And I would like to give honorable mentions to other Eastern civilizations such as the Chinese and the Koreans.

Ayurveda has been developed and evolved primarily in Ancient India. However, the Chinese and the Koreans, along with the Japanese, had made significant contributions to this system.

Oh wait, did I introduce myself? Oops, my bad. I'm Lakshmi, hailing from Southern India. I would like to take you through a detailed journey through the Ayurvedic realm, especially keeping depression and anxiety issues in mind. Why? Well, I've suffered from both these issues myself, and you guessed it right, Ayurveda had helped me cope and defeat those horrible mental health issues.

You know, I still remember that day. Oh, I'm talking about the day I had my first menstrual cramps. But, at that time, I didn't know much about it, other than the terrible pain in my belly. And then the bleeding started, yeah, from you know where. Oh boy, I was scared to the core. If you're a woman, I am sure you could understand what I'm saying. The panic, the chaotic fear, and many more emotions.

Mom took just a couple of minutes to figure out what's going on. It was exciting and nervous at the same time. More nervous, I must say.

Pretty normal, you must be thinking, right? Well, here comes the worst part. After three months, I've been diagnosed with PCOS! And those three months were the dreadful of my whole existence on this little blue planet. I put on a lot of weight, I started to lose hair, and my vaginal bleeding didn't know limits. Imagine going through all that at the age of 17!

Throughout this period, I had the lowest self-esteem someone could ever have. Okay, that might be a little exaggerating, but you got the point, right? I used to have cramps all over my lower body, making it very difficult to even sit. My hair, oh boy, that's a whole different story. I lost so much hair; you could even make a hair extension out of it. And the worst part, I used to bleed all the time, for which I had to take blood transfusions quite often.

After going through all these physical health conditions, I developed several mental health issues. Domino effect, eh! Who wouldn't be depressed when they put on a lot of weight, lose hair, and have cramps all day, every day?

I couldn't do anything other than lay in bed throughout the day and night. And there came my anxiety and depression. I felt like giving up on life. I felt like there's no one to save me, or should I say, nothing to save me? I tried a lot of things. Allopathy, the usual rescue for many people. Didn't work! Homeopathy forget about it.

When I was almost giving up, my granny suggested I go the Ayurvedic way. Boy, was she an angel! But, in hindsight, I should've considered it much earlier. Why? Well, it's the OG health system in our country for the last 5,000 years or even earlier. And, here I was, trying everything else and almost gave up with despair and hopelessness in my mind.

If you're feeling sorry for me, thank you for being empathetic. But this whole fiasco had helped in the bigger picture. Well, it made me stronger, taught me to toughen up in life and face my demons, both physical and psychological. After defeating my mental health issues, as well as physical ones, I'd like to help you guys too. I want you all to be healthy, especially by following a complete system of natural diet and lifestyle, which we lovingly call Ayurveda! So, buckle up, as I'm going to take you through a very detailed guide, which includes some science, some tips, and some serious health advice.

I've written this book to provide research and fact-based solutions. So, it's safe to say that you'll be reading about the science behind this amazing health system. I don't want to just give you lectures on how to do something. Rather, I would like to explain the Whys and Hows so that you can have a complete understanding of the problems and solutions as well.

Ayurveda, the ancient system of healing science, has its deep roots from India dating back to 5000 years and is a natural and holistic medicinal system. Ayurveda is hailed as the "mother of all healing." In Sanskrit, Ayurveda is AYUR, meaning life, and VEDA, meaning science hence said the science of life. As per Ayurveda, to achieve good health, one must be aware of all aspects of life.

Ayurveda is the world's oldest health science, from which Chinese, western medicine, and herbal medicine took birth. It believes that prevention is better than cure and focuses mainly on preventing disease, and when disease occurs, it eliminates from its root cause, rather than focusing just on symptoms. Allopathic medicine focuses on subsiding symptoms and managing the disease.

Some interesting facts:

1. You don't have to be an herbivore to practice Ayurveda. It's not a vegetarian philosophy.

2. During 300 BCE, an Ayurvedic scholar named Charaka used cannabis and opium poppy as potential painkillers since analgesics were not available. The use of it as an anesthetic and for sedation during surgeries are also mentioned in his book Charaka Samhita.

3. Ghee was known to cure nervous system disorders instantly. Every Indian household stores ghee in large vessels and passed it on to generations for the same.

4. Even before the invention of the microscope, 3000 years ago, Ayurveda knew anemia is caused by iron deficiency, and marasmus is treated by consuming liver and meat.

5. Did you know that tongue scraping and oil pulling were part of ayurvedic morning rituals? Tongue scraping with a copper scraper, due to its antibacterial properties, and the use of sesame oil for oil pulling to remove toxins (used as a mouth wash) are Ayurvedic techniques for oral hygiene.

How Does Ayurveda Work?

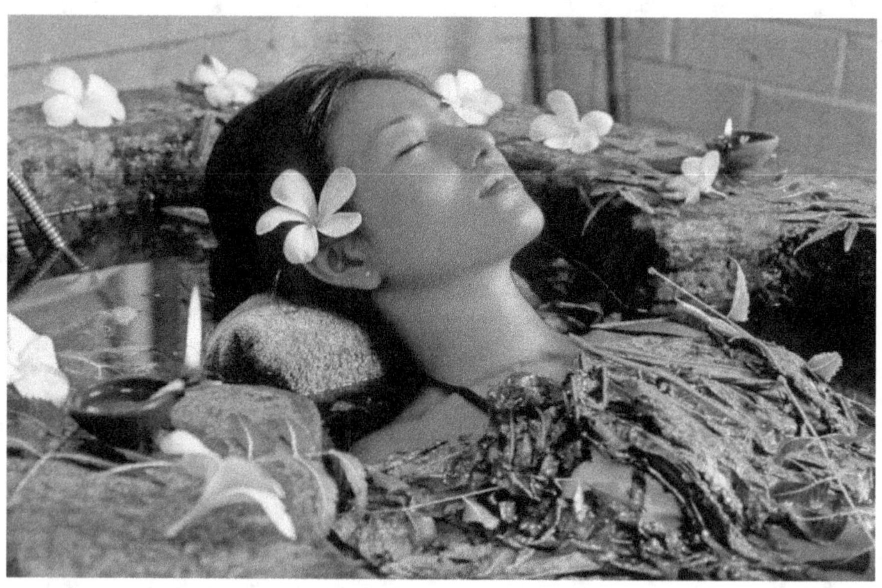

Ayurveda believes in the close association among man, the universe as well as the flow of cosmic energy in diverse forms within living and nonliving things. There is a Sanskrit saying based on two principle objectives of Ayurveda.

"Swasthasya swasthya samrakshanam athurasya vikaraprasamam."

"Swasthasya swasthya samrakshanam" means to prong life

and promote perfect health (adding years to life).

"Athurasya vikaraprasamam" means to completely eradicate disease and dysfunction of the body.

In Ayurveda, disease is a byproduct caused due to an imbalance or the stress in person's consciousness. The objective of Ayurveda is to maintain the health of a healthy person, to cure the health issues of a diseased person, to live gracefully and harmoniously in the balance of body, mind, spirit, and environment. It focuses on curing illness as well as prevention and promotion of health in a healthy individual.

Ayurveda with natural therapies and lifestyle changes helps regain lost balance. Ayurvedic therapies are typically based on complex herbal compounds, minerals, and metal substances under the influence of Indian alchemy or rasa shastra. Therapy includes an internal purification process, customized diet, herbal remedies and massage therapy, yoga, and meditation. Ancient Ayurveda texts also taught surgical techniques like rhinoplasty, kidney stone extractions, extraction of foreign objects, and suture placements.

Ayurvedic science has been widely adopted by western

medicine. The universal interconnections, prakruthi, that is the body's constitution, and doshas are life forces; these are the foundations of ayurvedic medicine. The goal is to eliminate impurities from the body and reduce symptoms, boost your immunity, and increase resistance to disease, reduce stress, and amplify harmony in life. Herbs are plants, spices, and oils that are used widely in ayurvedic treatment.

Ayurveda uses various methods for assessing health. The ayurvedic practitioner evaluates illness with key signs and symptoms in relation to its origin and root cause that led to an imbalance. Ayurveda believes that each one of us is unique, and we respond in our own way; we all have our strengths and weakness. Therapy is considered according to a patient's suitability for each unique individual. By interacting with a patient, questioning, patient's history, observation, and physical examination, they come to a conclusion.

They follow Basic methods like checking pulse, tongue, eyes, gait, physical appearance, voice during the examination. Palliative care, cleansing, when done appropriately, can keep imbalance at bay. Lifestyle changes, following strict dietary habits that have been suggested to you, and use of herbal medicine, cleansing programs like panchakarma helps the body to get rid of toxins and benefit from all these methods. The body, mind, and spirit are all addressed in Ayurveda. Through the wisdom of Ayurveda and its insights, experience. It is a gift to us with the vast wealth of data on the correlation between factors causing disease and its aftermath.

Techniques Employed in the Practice of Ayurveda

Dietary changes and mindfulness

Herbal medicine including herbs, metals, and minerals in the form of herbal powder, tablets, pellets.

Acupuncture

Massage

Meditation

Pranayama/ breathing exercise

Panchakarma/ five actions

Sound therapy - mantras

Yoga

Dietary Changes and Mindfulness

It promotes both mind and body. Ayurveda suggests eating specific foods based on your dominant dosha and achieves an inner balance among all three doshas. Ayurveda focuses on consuming unprocessed foods. One should practice mindful eating for better health.

Mindful eating is a technique of you having control over what you eat. In a fast-paced world full of gadgets, we are easily distracted and do not appreciate food eating became a mindless act. You will be able to recognize differences in physical hungry, cravings, emotional hunger, and fullness cues. It enhances self-control. One can achieve mindful eating by practicing eating slowly and chew thoroughly, eat in silence, and avoid distractions from gadgets. Feel the food by eating with the presence of mind. Stop eating once you are full. Eat consciously ask yourself if you are really hungry and healthy food.

Herbal Medicine

The herbal medicine includes herbs, metals, minerals in the form of herbal powder tablets, pellets. Herbal medicine is the use of plants to treat disease and enhance general health and wellbeing. Since the evolution of mankind on earth, humans have been dependent on plant resources. According to the World health organization, the report stated that over 80% of the world's population depends on plant-based medicine for their primary health care needs. The use of medicinal plants is cited in the Rig Veda and Charak Samhita, which says the Himalayas are the finest habitat for medicinal herbs.

At the earliest, Historic records of medicinal herbs were found during the Sumerian civilization, with hundreds of medicinal plants including opium poppy. It was also used for insomnia to induce sleep and relieve bowel-related issues.

The bark of willow trees and myrtle plants contain salicylic acid, which is an active metabolite of aspirin. Aspirin contains salicylate, and its use was recorded 4000 years ago. The great Hippocrates used willow bark for relieving pain and fevers.

Acupressure

Ayurvedic acupressure (marma therapy) is known to cure physical and mental issues. According to Ayurveda, the human body has 107 marma points; marma points are energy points where joints, muscle, bones, veins, and ligaments meet. They not only help in stimulation, circulation, improving mental and emotional stability but are meeting points of pain, weakness. Acupressure works best in allergies, migraine, PMS, chronic pain in the knees, neck, back, insomnia, anxiety, and depression.

Massage

Ayurvedic massage - it opens energy channels letting current flow freely to release energy. There are three movements involved in massage, strong pressure, delicate stroking, kneading the small muscles, thumb, and forefinger. Oil is applied in a direction that will help ease tension on the heart and activate the parasympathetic nervous system; this system conserves energy by reducing heart rate and increasing activity in the digestive system.

Meditation

Meditation is focusing the mind on one thought. Studies on meditators with 50-year-old brains had an equal amount of grey matter in the prefrontal cortex that 20 years old normally has. A 50-year-old has the same memory and decision-making abilities too. By meditating, our brain goes into an alpha wave pattern (resting phase) that is 'the power of now' being in the present. It helps us with a clear thought process, attentive mind, and achieve calmness and mental coordination. These waves are dominant in a meditative state and when thoughts flow quietly. Increase your serotonin- the happy hormone, creativity, intuition, memory, and retention, decrease your anxiety, stress, blood pressure, blood lactate, and tension related pain disorders.

Breathing Exercises

Pranayama/ breathing exercise - it's a practice of controlling breathing in yoga. Ancient sages in India knew those breathing techniques which are simpler to practice but had great potential to relax the body and mind. Pranayama can be practiced at any time of the day with an empty stomach.

1. Bhramari pranayama (bee breathing) - it's a boon for

hypertensive patients.

2. Kapal bhati pranayama (skull shining breathing) - helps in detoxification and unblocking the energy channels.

3. Bhastrika pranayama (bellows breath) - three rounds of this will rave-up your energy levels.

4. Nadi shodhan pranayama (alternate nostril breathing) - nine rounds of this technique and then 10 minutes of meditation calms and brings harmony among cerebral hemispheres, keeping neurological disorders at bay.

Panchakarma

Panchakarma/ five actions - Panchakarma is a method of elimination and intense detoxification of the body and balance three doshas. Panchakarma has five procedures for purification- vomiting (Vamana), Purgation(Virechana), Decoction enema (Niroohavasti), instillation of medicine through nostrils (Nasya), and oil enema (Anuvasanavasti). These procedures target causes and deep-rooted doshic imbalances.

Sound Therapy

Sound therapy - mantras - We all have come across ads of sound therapy apps while scrolling through Instagram. Sound therapy apps are a big thing of the 21st century, all thanks to our stressful life for giving us stress, anxiety, depression, and insomnia; millions of us are seeking peace and calmness. The good thing is they work. Mantra (sound) is the phonetic expression of the supreme reality. A mantra is a phonetic expression, a potent force composed of particular letters arranged in a specific sequence of sounds. Mantra is used to attain divine and mundane in nature. Scientists claim that chanting mantra rhythmically generates neurolinguistic effects that decrease anxiety and motivate us.

In patients suffering from Alzheimer's disease, their memories are often preserved because the key brain parts that preserve memories are linked to musical memory are relatively undamaged.

Yoga

Yoga is so popular around the globe that its popularity has led to the discovery of hybrid yogas like beer yoga, snow yoga, color yoga, themed yoga, hike yoga. This is a golden age of yoga, but the practice of yoga started thousand years ago and is hailed for its physical and mental benefits that are quite promising. So roll your mat and discover this beauty. Yoga improves alertness by enhancing the autonomic nervous system, so you will stay focused and energized without using harmful energy drinks.

The Fundamentals of Ayurvedic Healing

The main principle of Ayurveda states that the mind and body are connected, and the mind has the power to heal and transform a person's whole being. The philosophy of Ayurveda is based on the relation between microcosm and macrocosm involving five basic elements (pancha mahabhutha) space, air, fire, water, earth, three dynamic principles similar to humors (dosha) vata, pitta, kapha, seven types of tissues(dhatus) blood, fat, plasma, muscle, bone, reproductive fluids and bone marrow and many other unique concepts. Ayurveda is based on the belief that good health is achieved when a person achieves a balance among the mind, body, and spirit. We reflect the environments we are surrounded by, and with awareness, we transform our mind and body. Life in Ayurveda is perceived as the union of the body, senses, mind, and spirit. The concept of prakriti or nature has a pivotal role in Ayurveda treatments.

The Three Principle Energies

Ayurveda believes that pancha mahabhutas manifest in our body as three humors/tridoshas known as vata, pitta, and kapha. These three doshas regulate the creation, supporting, destruction, absorption, and excretion.

Three forces are vital to the concept of Ayurveda. These are the vata, pitta, and kapha.

1. Vata dosha, in which air and space elements dominate

2. Pitta dosha, in which the fire elements dominate

3. Kapha dosha, in which the earth and water elements dominate

Vata is viewed as wind, and it regulates the central nervous system. Whereas pitta is viewed as the sun, which is the source of energy and connected to the digestive system and biochemical processes, lastly kapha is viewed as earth and controls the cell regeneration and balance in the body's tissue fluids and muscular tone of the body. They circulate through the body and have an impact on the normal functioning of the body. They have effects on our food preferences and digestion and shape of the body, and finally the temperament of a person's mind and emotions. Unhealthy diet, muted emotions, lack of physical and mental exercise disturb one's doshic balance. Ayurveda believes in achieving perfect harmony by maintaining balance in doshas for optimum health.

Prakruthi

The concept of prakruti and tridhosahs being core philosophies of Ayurveda, prakruti explains a person's dosha and its composition and suggests each person's susceptibility to a particular dosha. Benefits of prakruthi not only include customized medicine and treatment but also customized prevention. It's worth bearing in mind that evidence connecting the core concepts like tridosha and prakruthi concerning metabolic pathways, chronic disease, and various genotypes have surfaced lately. Such evidence shed light on the universality of ayurvedic concepts as well as their clear linkage with concepts in modern science.

Ayurveda as a Complementary Healing System

Ayurveda is undoubtedly more effective than allopathic treatment in most of the longstanding health problems. However, modern medicines can relieve us quickly from disease but are quite expensive and come with an array of side effects. In recent times, fear of toxicity of allopathic drugs and unaffordability of health care system has made people seek alternative health systems like Ayurveda as a complementary healing system for chronic disease. An interesting fact is that Ayurveda recommends using a cooper utensil to purify water. Since copper has antibacterial effects and can prevent waterborne disease. Copper has antibacterial against Diarrheagenic bacteria like Vibrio cholera, Shigella flexneri, and enterotoxigenic bacteria like E Coli, enteropathogenic bacteria like salmonella enteric Typhi, E Coli, salmonella paratyphi is scientifically approved.

Health conditions like diabetes, arthritis, asthma, digestive disorders, and neurodegenerative disorders like Parkinson's disease, Alzheimer's disease, Huntington's disease are some problems Ayurveda is best sought for. Here is some evidence where Ayurveda performed better than modern medicine, especially in the case of chronic diseases. Problems that

Ayurveda can successfully combat are asthma, allergies, eczema, digestive disorders, osteoarthritis, rheumatoid arthritis, diabetes.

Ayurveda for Osteoarthritis

A study from 2013 conducted clinical trials in 440 people with knee osteoarthritis compared the efficiency of two ayurvedic formulations of natural glucosamine sulfate from plant extracts against drug celecoxib. All of them showed similar effects in relieving pain and function improvement.

Ayurveda for Rheumatoid Arthritis

A small pilot study funded by NCCIH with 43 patients suffering from rheumatoid arthritis was conducted to find out the efficiency of conventional drug methotrexate and ayurvedic medicine that had 40 herbal compounds found out that both had similar effects.

Ayurveda for Type 2 Diabetes

A small short-term clinical trial that had 89 patients, including both men and women suffering from type 2 diabetes, sought effective help from five herbs.

Ayurveda for Ulcerative Colitis

Studies conducted on turmeric, a spice often used in most of the Ayurvedic preparations, may help with ulcerative colitis; a study published in 2005 had 10 participants, and a study published in 2006 had 89 participants.

Ayurveda for Asthma

The use of herbs that have antiasthmatic, bronchodilator, and antihistamine properties. Herbs like holy basil, argemone Mexicana, cassia sophora, Euphorbia hirta, aka asthma weed, piper betel help people with asthma.

History, Origin, and Decline of Ayurveda

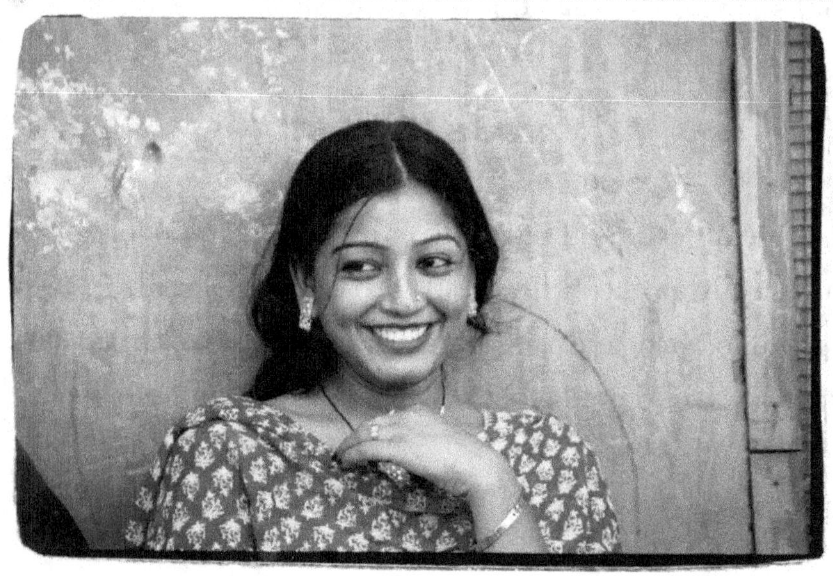

Ayurveda has evolved over the decades. They orally passed ayurvedic knowledge for generations through the lineage of sages, and eventually, it became the leading medical system in India. Ayurveda flourished in Ancient India, grew in harmony with Unani medicine in Medieval India but was turned down during British rule. It was suppressed in India during British colonial rule. In 1833, the East India company closed and banned all ayurvedic colleges. During the British rule, that system was a cloak and dagger operation but was still practiced in rural areas. It was claimed as the poor man's medicine, whereas modern medicine was unaffordable and unavailable. After a time, Ayurveda resurfaced and spread far and wide and into other civilizations worldwide.

In India, Ayurveda is contemplated as a form of medical care, equivalent to modern medicine, traditional Chinese medicine, naturopathy, and homeopathy. Practitioners of Ayurveda in India undergo state-recognized, institutionalized training India has over 400,000 registered Ayurveda practitioners; the ayurvedic education, practice, and its quality is regulated by the government of India. With high professional competence and respect to traditional countries like Germany, Italy, Hungary, Switzerland, the United States are correctly practicing Ayurveda. Ayurveda had a deep-rooted effect on Tibetan medicine (Sowa-rigpa medicine), traditional Chinese medicine, conventional medicines of Persia, Egypt, Greece, Rome, and Indonesia were also taken from Ayurveda.

Ayurveda has a long history, and its basic principles may be valid even today. The spirit of any science is a continuous hunt and a thirst for new knowledge through research, evolution, and newer applications. The mode of manifestation of the disease has changed. Man-made developments have changed the geo-climatic environment and stressed our plants, animals, and microbes, and put them on the verge of extinction. The human race has made headway in their behavior, lifestyle, and genetics.

Vedas

Vedas are four sacred texts. Ayurveda dates back to the Vedic era and was written 5000 years ago in Sanskrit in these sacred texts. They are named as the Rig Veda during 3000-2500 BCE and Yajur Veda, Sam Veda, and Atharva Veda during 1200-1000 BCE. Most of the information on health and diseases are cited in Atharva Veda. Rig Veda has information on diseases and medicinal plants.

Texts in Ayurveda

The knowledge of Ayurveda was taught orally from accomplished masters to their disciples and then to human physicians in India. Some of this knowledge was all set to be jotted down a few thousand years ago, but most of it was obscured.

The oldest known texts on Ayurveda are the Charaka Samhita, Sushruta Samhita (400BC- 200 AD), and ashtanga hrudhaya. The lesser three classics of Ayurveda are sharangadhara Samhita, bhava Prakasha, and Madhava nidanam(800AD). Ayurveda was open to new ideas, principles, and knowledge for continuous progress. Modernity is the result of the evolution of traditions and not a static entity. Just in case if there had been the availability of devices like thermometers or electronic microscopes, do you think our ayurvedic scholars would be ignorant towards using them. No, they would be happy to see ayurvedic science progressing.

Charaka Samhita

Charaka Samhita, a most popular book in Ayurveda till today written by Agnivesha, later renamed Charaka. Probably, there won't be any ayurvedic physician who has not studied Charaka. The work has detailed medical information on diseases from facts, diagnosis, treatments, and medicines. It also detailed the medicinal value and qualities of over 10,000 herbal plants. Book also had 84 alcoholic preparations and their medicinal value. Importance of hygiene, diet, prevention. The importance of medical education is also mentioned.

Sushruta Samhita

Sushruta Samhita, authored by Sushruta, explains the concept and practice of surgery in Ayurveda. It is composed of 184 chapters and presents 1120 health conditions, 300 types of operations that require 42 different surgical procedures,121 instruments that are used for practice, and 650 kinds of medicine derived from plants, minerals, and animals. This book deals with general aspects, health issues, and treatment. It described the anatomy of eyes in a way that all the complex things are also dealt with, as in contemporary science. It Estimated that 72 eye diseases of the iris and pupil are discussed, including invasive procedures for cataracts, preglaucomatic conditions, glaucoma, pink eye, pterygium, and cosmetic surgeries for the nose and ears like rhinoplasty and auroplasty have also been mentioned in the texts.

Ashtanga Hrudhya

Ashtanga hrudhya was a simplified version of ashtanga sangraha, a classic formed by Vagbhata. Its emphasis on kayachikitsa, the section of Ayurveda that focuses on internal medicine, doshas, and their subsections were presented in detail. Ashtanga sangraha is famous for its point of view in analytical classification arrangement Sant and presentation;

Vagbhata excels other writers for the same reason for that being most popular work than others among students and practitioners in down south of India. Vagbhata was the first author to have begun the syncretic schools and put all information together from all the branches of medicines within reach of single work. He divided it into eight parts (Astanga) and named as ashtanga hrudhya. The eight branches were general medicine, mental diseases, diseases of sensory organs, pediatrics, toxicology, surgery, gerontology, and aphrodisiac. Ayurveda is the only ancient science where geriatrics health care was a prime concern, and therapies for old age were mentioned. The branch of geriatrics focuses on rejuvenation and delay aging and geriatric degeneration and promote healthy longevity in old age.

Sharnagadhara Samhita

Sharnagadhara Samhita, written by Sharngadhara, flourished during the 11th century AD and explained pharmacological formulations used in panchakarma. In this book, it's depicted that the diagnosis of a person's health status is made through their pulse. Sarangadhara Samhita contains valuable definitions of technical terms, called paribhasa, and is very popular among practitioners all over the world for its use of handy prescriptions.

Bhava Prakasha

Bhavaprakasa, by Bhavamisra, is the last and mayhaps the best work of the medieval age. The term between the 10th till the 16th Century AD. is the extremely futile and dormant period in the literature of Ayurveda. Foreign invasions like British rule and internal turmoil lead to stagnation in Ayurveda. When Bhavamisra resumed the traditions of writing, he reviewed the developments of the medieval period and included various new diseases and drugs. He is the first author to refer to the disease, 'Phirangaroga,' which was apparently the technical name of syphilis. The word 'Phiranga' means foreigners, that is, the Portuguese in particular, Europeans in general, in many of the Indian languages. The term 'Phiranga Roga'or Portuguese disease came into use to describe syphilis, as the disease syphilis was the first well-recorded European outbreak that occurred in 1495 to have been brought to India by Europeans.

Madhava Nidanam

Madhava Nidanam, a diagnostic classic authored by Madhava, discussed toxicology and conditions of the nose, ears, throat, and diseases that involve women and children, providing over 5,000 signs and symptoms. In his book, he wrote about five aspects of diagnosis know as aetiological pentad (nidana panchaka). They are primary symptoms (purvarupa) and manifested symptoms (rupa), samprapti (pathogenesis), upasaya (therapeutic tests), and ashta vidha pareeksha (eight types of medical examinations). Rheumatoid arthritis was first explained in this.

These texts have the detailed effects of five elements found in the cosmic system - earth, water, air, fire, space have on individual systems and tell us the importance of keeping these elements balanced for a healthy and happy life. In Ayurveda, we are influenced by certain elements. This is because of their natural constitution or prakriti.

Scholars like Vagbhata and Sharangdhara have set out the 10- phasic sequential biological changes taking place during the 1st to 10th decades of life.

Ageing Decades Inherent Biolosses

0-10 Balya – Corpulence/strong

11-20 Vriddhi –Growth/elongation

21-30 Chhabi – Lusture/coquette

31-40 Medha- Intellect/comprehension

41-50 Twaka – Skin quality

51-60 Drishti – Vision Locomotion

61-70 Shukra – Virility

71-80 Vikrama – Physical Strength

81-90 Buddhi – Thinking

91-100 Karmendriya - Locomotion

These may be restored up to a workable extent by adopting age-specific rasayanas.

The Concepts of Ayurveda: Tridhoshic Theory

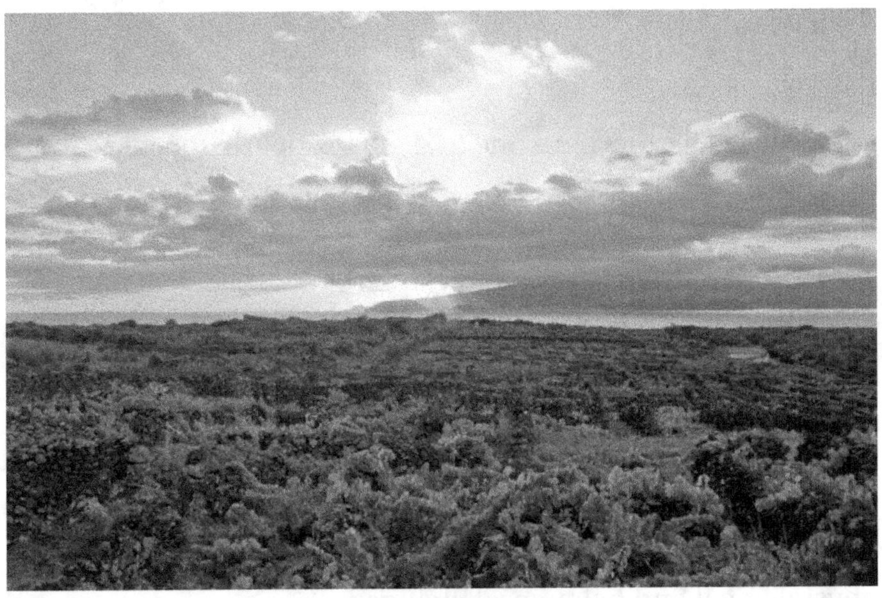

These forces actively alter a person's dietary habits and their thoughts and seasons. Changing our diets according to changes in the environment plays a crucial role in keeping us healthy. Identifying dosha composition will lead us to take measures to bring balance in their state. As your health demands, one has to juggle with doshas to poise them. They influence our likes and dislikes, appearance, our tendencies, and habits, our mental and emotional character. This constitution serves as a blueprint for optimal health.

Three situations in which doshas can be apparent are:

1. Ideal state is achieving a state of balance in all three doshas.

2. Increased state where one of dosha is in greater proportion to others.

3. Lastly, the decreased state is when one of the doshas is lesser than other doshas.

When there's an imbalance in the natural proportions of these doshas, it is known as vikruti. It can show symptoms in physiological and behavioral changes.

Vata Dosha

Vata is thought to be head of the three ayurvedic principles. It's known to be dynamic and the principle of mobility; it mostly regulates all activities of the body, be it mental, physical, or physiological.

Definition: Vata is made of air and ether components, controlling our nervous system and all the motions happening in our body. When Vata is imbalanced, we feel constipated, bloated, anxious, and encounter irregular periods.

Functions: It is responsible for prime involuntary activities like breathing, blinking eyes and heartbeat, blood circulation, lungs, diaphragm, and gastrointestinal tract and carries the function of an excretory system like the elimination of feces, urine, sweat, and menstruation. Ingestion, communication, heart function, orgasm, creativity and emotions, and sensory functions like hearing and touch. The nervous system functions like peristalsis and enzyme secretion, and all physical movements, exercise.

A person with Vata dosha where Vata is dominant may exhibit their imbalance through various symptoms:

General symptoms such as limpness, dizziness, dehydration, mental confusion, anxiety, cough, dry hair and dry skin, poor blood circulation, respiratory issues, feeling cold all the time, heart palpitations, hearing problems, loss of senses.

Some symptoms in the digestive system include loss of

appetite, discomfort after eating, low stomach acid, bloating gas, constipation, impaired nutrient assimilation from food.

Pelvic area symptoms like lack of menstruation, inability to orgasm, vaginal dryness, loss of sexual interest, amenorrhea, and infertility.

Some orthopedic issues like osteoporosis, arthritis.

Mental illness symptoms like anxiety, insomnia, flakiness, mood swings, dementia, lack of creativity, nervousness, mental instability, forgetfulness, fatigue, memory loss.

Rest is needed to balance your Vata; it is vibrant and zestful when in balance.

Vata Characteristics: Vatas can binge eat and not gain extra pounds. you have a hard time gaining weight and muscle mass even while overindulging. You are small-boned, and your joints seem to be cracking quite often. Do you fall under extremes, either tall or short, lots of legroom or no legroom? You tend to dry out like deserts and have dry bodies, dry skin, hair, and nails.

Brace yourself! You need braces to deal with your natural

crooked teeth and thin pale gums. You have thin skin, and raccoon eyes are just a few nights of sleep away. You don't sweat and often feel cold. You often experience back problems and have bony abnormalities, such as scoliosis or bunions.

You guys love to think outside the box and are extremely creative, and their subjects of interest are philosophy, literature, and spirituality. Like the characters in Gilmore girls, talking a mile a minute is your thing. Since you have a million things going on in your head. You are a flipflopper who have a restless energy and tend to overthink. More prone to nervous system issues like anxiety, nervousness, and panic attacks. If you relate to these things, then make sure to work on them.

Pitta Dosha

Definition: Pitta is composed of the fire and water elements, controlling our stomach and transformations within your body. When pitta is out of balance, you experience heartburn, overeating, anger, impatience, and other related issues.

Pitta is the fire element and is responsible for digestive fire.

Comprised of fire and water, it is fiery, sharp, creasy, fluid, and light, much like the fire and water.

Pitta is in charge of transformation in the body. It regulates body temperature through the chemical transformation of food. It promotes vitality and appetite. It is mostly in your belly, liver, lower intestines, spleen, blood, gallbladder. And is responsible for digestion, nutrient absorption, metabolism. Pitta helps our stomach to break down food with the help of digestive enzymes in the small intestine and pepsin and hydrochloric acid in your stomach. Furthermore, pitta is present as bile in your liver. Haemoglobin, the main protein that carries oxygen in the blood, has pitta within it. Pitta also manages your thirst, taste, vision, body temperature, the luster of skin and hair, food, and skin sensitivities.

People with pitta dosha are strong-willed, stubborn, and have strong leadership qualities. Pitta is also responsible for being intelligent, courageous, ambitious, and are determined. Now think of yourself and see if you fall into this category with such great qualities. If yes, then let me explain how you react when you are imbalanced. When pitta is imbalanced, it leads to anger and agitation. The body excretes excess pitta through sweat, which is a vital thing to release that additional pitta that's getting accumulated. So, next time when you work out, be proud that you are also detoxifying your body.

When pitta is imbalanced, you may experience general symptoms like feeling hot all the time, excessive sweating, and to make it even worse, that sweat is going to be foul-smelling; you might want to stock up on some deodorants. Baldness in early age and premature greying, hair problems are the worse they take a toll on your confidence, poor eye vision, excess bile that in turn shows up with yellow eyes and skin over the period, malfunctioning liver, photosensitivity are the symptoms you never want to have.

Digestive symptoms like burning disorders like hyperacidity, inflammation, acid reflux, ulcers, heartburn, and diarrhea.

Mental symptoms like anger, frustration, narcissism, competitiveness, stress, burnout, irritability, hatred, and impatience.

Pitta Characteristics: Physically, pittas are easy muscle gainers; few sessions of pumping iron are all you need to see the greatest gains. They are naturally athletic with medium-built bodies—not too strong and big, but not too small and weak. You tend to have greasier hair that's sad and droopy within no time after wash. Grey-headed hair or balding in your 30s with oily skin that often causes breakouts.

Your skin and hair have a reddish tint. You start to sweat buckets and become overheated and feel baked easily; you can't live without air-conditioning. You have a freckly face and are redheaded, which makes you stand out. Your face has moles that are signature marks. You are more prone to sunburns, rashes, rosacea, and psoriasis.

Mentally, pittas are very driven and have achievement-oriented leadership qualities, and work hard towards being successful. Business, law, finance, fitness, science interest you. You have perfectionist mentalities, organized minds and do well with structure. You are very dominating and compulsive when that drive becomes excessive. You can be controlling, demanding, and impatient with others.

You are prone to burnout and adrenal fatigue. You fall somewhere in the middle ground of vata-pitta or pitta-vata.

Kapha Dosha

Kapha is a combination of earth and water. It is strong,

sluggish, cold, greasy, gentle, dense, and fluid, just like earth and water.

Definition: Kapha controls our bone density and the whole structure of our body. When Kapha is out of balance, you experience heaviness, fatigue, water retention, depression, and other related issues.

Kapha is accountable for anabolism, the process of building the body, growth, and new cell regeneration and cell repair. It is in charge of body structure, bone density, and strength, stamina, fat regulation, fertility. It is found in your lungs, stomach, pancreas, lymphatic system, plasma, tongue, and nose, joint, and sinuses. Kapha is compared to earth for its functions in providing strength, support, and stability like our home earth. Kapha is known to maintain body resistance. Kapha dominated people are known to be thoughtful, calm, and composed. Kapha works as a lubricant and relieves friction between cells and organs. Present in your joints and muscles, making you physically strong to help you go on hiking or dancing even in your 70s.

All bodily fluids, such as saliva, mucus, and semen, are associated with kapha. Kapha also controls lubrication, cell repair and restoration, the structure and energy of the body, growth and stability, mucus and moisture, body mass and body fat, grounding, and nurturance, memory retention, giving nature and kindness.

When Kapha is imbalanced, you experience general symptoms like feeling cold all the time, clammy hands, weight gain, lethargy, mucus buildup, white-coated tongue, asthma, phlegm, infections, swelling, and water retention. Digestive system symptoms include slow metabolism, heaviness after meals, slow and sticky stools, and bloating. Symptoms of mental health issues include feeling lethargic depressed, lonely, sad, jealous, and lack of attachment.

Kapha Characteristics: Physically, kaphas have a very slow metabolism that you tend to put on weight just by thinking about food. You are hefty, large-framed, bigger boned with round faces and bodies. You are blessed with thick, lustrous hair and soft, smooth, supple skin, and perfect nails. You prefer dry, warm weather and cold hands and regulate their body temperature well. You are fond of deserts and have a sweet tooth.

Mentally, kaphas are very kind and humane. They tend to be responsible and thoughtful about things around them. You are accountable for human resources; you are a public person and interested in teaching, human resources, nursing, therapy, and service-based activities. You often put others before them and are people pleasers. You are calm and composed, peace-loving, but you are slow as snail resistant to change and are procrastinators. You are depressed souls and often dwell in the past; you tend to gain weight by depressed eating. Depression and overeating go hand in hand.

If you have a bit of the vata type, you are a kapha-vata or vata-kapha; if you are mixed with the pitta type, you are a kapha-pitta or pitta-kapha. It's extremely rare to be tridoshic, that is, to have balance among all three. But it is more likely that we have imbalances in all three.

Making Sense of the Doshas

Now that you have an idea about the doshas and have figured out where you stand Let's put some useful knowledge to bring to bear on doshic situations. This way, you'll be able to spot vatas, pittas, and kaphas in people around you, and let's try to fathom these doshas in-depth to make better sense of these doshas. I will make sure you learn specific imbalances associated with each dosha and put them right on track for healthful living. We are a combination of all three doshas in varying levels. In this hurry-scurry life, it's okay sometimes to have an imbalance concerning other doshas. There comes a moment in your life when You will most likely have imbalances with all three doshas and once in a while relate to another dosha when it's not your prime dosha.

Vata Types

Vatas are very impulsive, and your mind always throws up innovative ideas. You want to make things big and are always up for challenges. You cannot bear monotony in mind and want to try new things, boredom hits them easily of being at one place for too long and can sit still and are always wandering to do something instead of being ideal. You look into the bigger picture of things, which often others won't. Any visionary, artist, writer, a philosopher can be an example of data. Vata types are creative. Vatas thrive in creative careers like entertainment and business. Eminent personalities like Elon Musk, Steve Jobs, William Shakespeare, Christopher Nolan, Leonardo da Vinci, Jim Carrey, Uma Thurman, Steven Spielberg, Will Smith, and Quentin Tarantino fall into this category.

Physically, vatas wander like a vagabond; they move around a lot. You might have seen some of your friends or yourself not able to sit through a movie. Then they are vatas, shaking leg personality. You may often see yourself shaking legs and can't be still. Vatas look long and lean. You get cold easily, so you need to keep your environment warm; you tend to pace when you are thinking but not do well in a cubicle. You need your surroundings to constantly change to stay driven. You have countless things running in your mastermind, from showering genius ideas to beating a dead horse, persistent repetition of words and thoughts in your mind, analyzing baseless points, you are easily abstracted and inattentive. You stray from the subject. You sometimes act like you have (ADHD) attention deficit disorder. Things can sometimes go wrong with all this fuss over nothing. You will have a difficult time traveling, and you are nauseated the whole journey. To help you with this, you can sip warm ginger tea sweetened with brown sugar. You also have a sensitive digestive system, so it's healthy to eat warm food.

When you have a brain like a sieve, it's wise to do one thing at a time. Practicing meditation is a pipe dream. It gives you the heebie-jeebies, just sitting still. You are always in the foreseeable future. You should pull your wandering mind into the present. You worry about things that never happen. Did you know that about 85% of things we worry about never really happen? We all have vata moments in life - we all have things hanging in our heads, and on anxious seats, sometimes we are overwhelmed. And it's okay to feel this way at times. After all, we are in a vata-centric society. We all try to squeeze things all at once (walk and chew gum). This makes it extremely difficult to keep our eyes on the ball. You get bored easily due to your short attention span. When you sense all these things going on, it's extremely important to let your hair down for once and calm your vatas. You are all over the place and experience mood swings. You are extremely sensitive to your surroundings and develop a dislike towards certain sounds, and it upsets you. If you think you fall into this category, you must work on pacifying your vata. You are more at the stake of feeling the ill effects

Here's a snapshot of Vata types:

Vata mind: Creative

Vata body: Lean

Vata obstacle: Sticking to one idea

Vata imbalance: Anxiety, digestive trouble

Pitta Types

Mentally, pitta types are ambitious and hard-working. They are very focused and like to do one thing at a time efficiently. They possess strong leadership qualities and do well in managing things. They have minds that are quite organized and work on schedule, and they comply with the deadlines.

To finish the task, they would burn the candle at both ends. Sportspersons, business tycoons, managers, financial analysts, lawyers will fall into this category. Some people who are pitta types are the great boxer, Muhammad Ali, shooting guard Kobe Bryant and wisest investor warren Buffett, presidents Donald Trump, Franklin Roosevelt, Brad Pitt, Madonna. Pittas excel in being Professional athletes and politicians. Pittas have a great deal of fire energy within them that needs to be released. Physically, pittas need a good workout, and you love to physically exhaust their bodies and energy within them that needs to be released. You love to stay physically active and drain their bodies and use their muscle. You are sportive and are good athletes, do well in sports, military camps, marathons and at competitions. You love to trek, cycle, swim, run; basically, you are a triathlon. For you, this is more about personal goals than the competition.

Pittas are angry birds and are impatient. They heat up quickly, and this can be obvious with hot temperatures or hot in anger. Pittas are up in arms when things don't go their way. You are annoyed when others take too long to perform the task. Pittas except for everyone around them to work and put as much effort as they do. You set their standards high and want everyone to do the same One frequent stumbling block for pittas is that all the fire in their bodies will transfer into the fire in their minds making them angry birds. Pittas can be intimidating and give a hard time to people working under them. You are like a ball of fire; the fire they carry within themselves begins to burn them. You have a bundle of energy that sometimes surpasses their limits. You are more prone to burnout from working restlessly. You don't appreciate relaxing and have difficult times taking things easily when things don't go as per your plan. You stress out, and their mental soundness is compromised, making them more vulnerable to adrenal fatigue; these things may jeopardize your mental health. The biggest task for you is to calm down and take things slowly. Much like drug addiction, you deal with work addiction, and you love being a work addict. Finishing tasks and achievements can make you feel high. You tend to do one after other tasks and on a roll due to that pitta energy; however, if you continue at this pace without rest, no wonder!

Your brain hurts, you are overtiring your mind, and it leads to breakdown. You should stop beating your brains out. It's important to relax and practice some self-care and take care of your mental health and body. After all, that's the only place you live in. Wrap your brain around things that are your favorite. Recharge it and make a grand comeback. Since you are swamped with work, you constantly fear missing something important. This fear will stop us from thinking logically and analyzing things. So, find out what is the need of the hour and try to minimize your workload, and use your headspace wisely. Calm your brain that's been an active volcano for a long time.

Simply turn off alerts from your emails and switching off your phone, or activate your do not disturb mode. By doing these, you reduce your cognitive load. Use cognitive boosters such as plant-based, fresh and unprocessed foods. Increasing your cerebral blood flow for best thinking rewire your brain by increasing the level of physical activity; this will supply your brain with extra oxygen and nutrients. Spend on unfocused thinking for 20 minutes daily, get up for a good stretch with yoga, or grab a glass of detox drink and go for a walk. Your life has always been about finishing things from the to-do list and doing projects at a stretch.

For you, time is money. You don't stop, so cultivating a few of those habits can reboot and energize your brain to go the extra mile for the next chunk of work. It helps you maintain cognitive stamina across the day and improves your sleep cycles. These will fire up your brain; trust me when I say this, it's going to change your life. This is all about pitta moments. If you are someone who likes to have a lot on your plate, then you would lose your friends and loved ones. You lack time for them. Pitta types need to slow down and take it easy.

Pittas have a strong digestive fire; they can eat foods that are raw and cold without worrying about digestive problems. However, it's best to avoid peppery foods that increase your fire. Foods like cucumber, mint, and coconut water can be soothing for you.

Here's a snapshot of Pitta types:

Pitta mind: Ambitious

Pitta body: Athletic

Pitta obstacle: Burnout

Pitta imbalance: Anger, heartburn

Kapha Types

Mentally, kaphas are peace-loving, grounded, calm, and composed. You are patient and do work at a snail's pace, but a good thing is that you do the work thoroughly. You are easy-going and generous; by no means your generosity is limited. You care for people around you and have no expectations in return. You put others before you, you are optimistic, and kindness is your strength. Kapha types have humility. Kapha types are altruistic. You give without hoping for anything in return as compensation for the good deeds you make. You are idealistic. You set some principles in life, which you will follow no matter what. You have certain things to follow on how to be a responsible citizen, and you strive to achieve them till the end.

You want to make this world a better place, you don't stop giving your money, time, and anything that it takes to make this world a better place. You go out of your way to please your loved ones without any hesitation. You are extremely loyal, and trust is your major quality. You are extremely loyal, and people place confidence in you. Your friendships and relationships are long-lasting than usual. Kaphas are extremely reliable and trustworthy whom one can count on. You are extremely patient even when things don't go their way; you don't complain even in the toughest times or while accomplishing a tough task.

With patience, they develop self-control, and being patient for them means not giving up on things easily without trying. You are great listeners and good at analyzing and counseling. Kaphas are empathizers. They are sensible and try to see other problems being in their shoes. You are a magnet to people's problems. You take your hobbies seriously and keep your hands working on them. Kaphas love knitting, sewing, and handicrafts. You enjoy cooking and love to try new dishes, and you love to feed your loved ones with that food; they also like gardening and like to grow their food. Above our life, don't we all love a steadfast friend? If you have come across friends who always put other's needs before theirs, like the saying, "a friend in need is a friend indeed," then he or she is a kapha. When imbalanced, kaphas binge eat, and do not move their body, put on weight easily, and end up being diabetic. Kaphas just need food and sleep and nothing else. Kaphas love to rest. Kaphas are clinophiles and love to sleep a lot; the mere sight of their beds makes them happy. They love anything sweet, sour, and salty. Kaphas are moist, cold, oily, soft skin and heart, dull, static, smooth, dense, long eyelashes, and thick brows.

Foods that are spicy and hot are a good choice for you. You may avoid foods like red meat, dairy products, and fried foods. You have a sweet tooth and crave deserts after each meal.

Some famous people who are kapha types are Ellen DeGeneres, Oprah Winfrey, Jimmy Kimmel, and Rachel Ray. Kaphas possess nurturing qualities; they make good parents. They work as caregivers, nurses, and teachers. Nobel professionals like doctors, hospital workers, therapists, nursing staff fall under this type. Kaphas are generous, kind, and compassionate. They want to help people. People with these traits being in these particular professions can make this world a lot better place. Teaching is a very humanistic profession. A good teacher can be a role model and can teach morals and human values to students.

Physically, kaphas are often blessed with big eyes, full lips, and look like dolls gifted with beautiful angelic voices, like Adele, Beyonce. Actors like George Clooney, Angelina Jolie come under this class. They are naturally curvy; they have the greater glyph of stamina of all three doshas. However, when they are out of balance, they allow their sedentary nature to take over, and they lack exercise, causing them to feel heavier and gain weight. Socialization can help improve your mental and emotional health. It promotes purpose and increases the quality of life.

This is why they need to stay active to keep them in balance. Kaphas need good exercise. You should be doing cardio, lifting weights, break out in a sweat. Kaphas are so busy keeping everyone around them happy that they often forget to take care of themselves. You are all ears for other people's problems but have a hard time voicing your own.

You are in smiles and always cheerful, try to put a smile on others and keep them happy, but deep down, they bare sadness. You feel you are alone in this world and feel you lack a support system. You support everyone around you, but you have no one to take care of you. And face everything by yourself. You will never show your sadness. You tend to put a brave front and step out in a smile and feign happiness. So that you won't be questioned about their sadness or the state of mind they are currently in. Sometimes, they feel like not showing their emotions due to the fear of being ridiculed and pitied.

We all know that there's a strong correlation between overeating and depression. Due to prolonged sadness, kaphas tend to overeat and gain weight. Depression triggers overeating as a coping mechanism for emotional relief. Longstanding sorrow keeps growing, and you feel numb, emotionally distanced, and lack interest in socializing and hold things for yourself; they don't want to bother others with their problems. You are overwhelmed with grief. And you become lethargic and put on weight. You need to start making small changes one at a time into leading a more active life and making conscious decisions, growing and evolving in life. Once you set your mind in motion, you will have brainstorming ideas coming your way. You will start to embrace life when slowly, everything will fall back into place.

We may all have been there; nothing in this world excited us anymore. We didn't have anyone around us who would understand us; getting out of bed was a real challenge. Some days the world wears you down. Due to heaviness, you have a tough time getting out of your comfort zone. But that's okay times like these happen to everyone, and it's important to bounce back. Wake up before the sun is out, and you will see yourself being more focused and productive. You will sport a clear calmer mind in bustling morning energy that keeps you motivated. Take a deep breath, pick yourself up, and chalk out your plan, start all over again and win your life.

Here's a snapshot of Kapha types:

Kapha mind: Peaceful

Kapha body: Rounded

Kapha obstacle: Putting others before self

Kapha imbalance: Depression, weight gain

Traits of the Three Doshas

Characteristic	Vata	Pitta	Kapha
Body frame	Small frame	Medium frame	Large frame
Physique and Musculature	Feeble	Moderately built	Well built
Skin	Dry, Dull, and chapped skin	Soft, smooth, thin and has birthmarks, prone to acne, and freckly skin	Even skin, firm, clean and clear skin tone
Hair	Dry and frizzy,	Thin, sparse,	Thick,

	thin, with split ends	oily, premature greying	lustrous hair, smooth in texture
Body weight	Uncooperative	Unstable	Tendency to be obese
Food habits and bowel movements	Frequent consumption variable, and irregular movements	Consume a lot of food and drink plenty of water	Stable dietary habits and low digestive capacity
Mobility and physical exercise	Exorbitant mobility and brisk	Moderate mobility	Lesser mobility and slow
Tolerance for changes in seasonal weather	Sensitive to Cold	Sensitive to Heat	They Tolerate both heat and cold
Resistance to disease and the ability to heal	Poor prognosis	Good prognosis	Excellent prognosis
Detoxification of toxins	Moderate	Rapid	Inadequate

Communication skills	Talkative and sociable	Good analytical abilities and Sharp communication skills	Less vocal but are great at communic ating
Capability to initiating new things	Enthusiastic, flexible, and Quick initiators	Moderate initiators once realized	Slow initiators
Memory	Clever and grasp promptly but lack retention	Average grasping power and retention	Grasp slowly but have good retention
Aging	Age fast	Age Moderately	Age Slowly
Disease Susceptibility and Prognosis	Vulnerable to Developmental and neurological diseases like Dementia, mobility, speech disorders, and arrhythmias	More prone to skin diseases and ulcers	Prone to be obese, diabetic

Personality Description of Three Doshas

Vata Dosha	Pitta Dosha	Kapha Dosha
Lean and fragile body and dull skin, fine hair	Moderately built and muscular	They have Strong frame and dense bones
Dynamic and energetic	Kind and generous	Calm and composed, slow to react
Light-hearted and quite expressive	Stubborn and have a powerful will and are passionate leaders	Loving, caring, and easy-going personality
Highly innovative, they are flexible in behavior and making decisions and have fluctuating mood	Straight forward and ready to take charge	They are stable and thoughtful. Tend to move slowly and steadily

Branches of Ayurveda

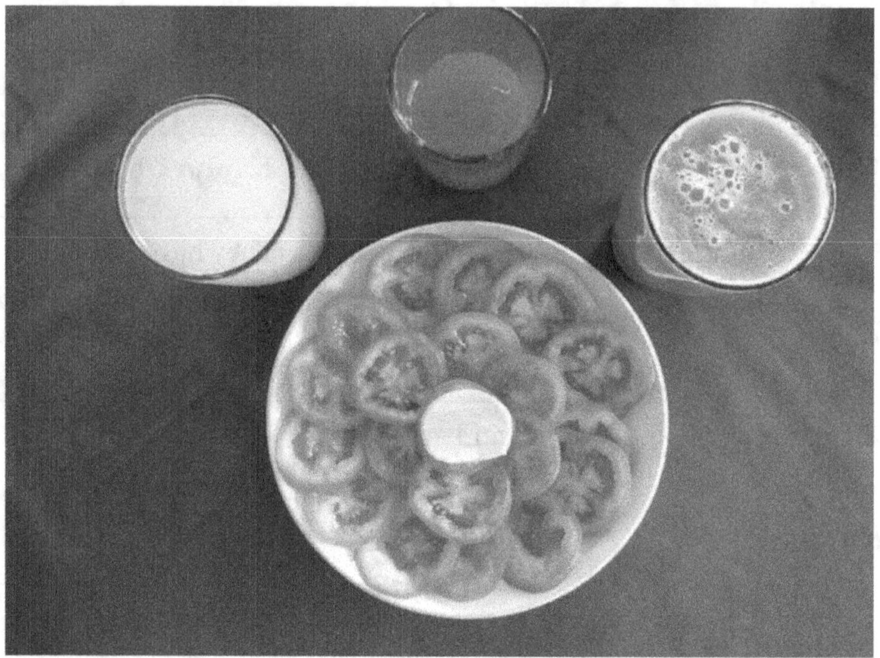

Eight elements in ayurvedic medicine are collectively called ashtang Ayurveda.

Kayachikitsa, or internal medicine - focuses on the body's digestive system and metabolism. Although this branch focuses on the overall treatment of the entire body. Procedures can be carried out both internally and externally. Taking medicines orally, and applying lotions, oils, creams are part of this treatment.

Baala chikitsa or pediatrics - this branch focuses on disease and sickness in infants, children, and adolescents, also deals with pre and postnatal care. Ayurvedic practitioners keep in mind that children cannot explain what they are going through and prescribe medicines accordingly, which is pleasant on the palate.

Graha chikitsa or psychiatry - this branch deals with problems and diseases of the mind. Treating our mind includes various ways like adding herbs that help the mind calm. Yoga, pranayama, and chanting mantras. Which is called mantra chikitsa.

Urdhyaanga chikitsa- deals with health issues in the upper part of the body, includes the head, ear, nose, eye, throat. It is concerned with all problems in and around the head.

Shalyaroga chikitsa or surgery - concerned with surgical procedures. It tells the use of surgical devices such as scalpels and scissors.

Damstra chikitsa or toxicology - this branch deals with the study to prevent and cure the effects of toxins and poisons in the body, food, and environment.

Jara chikitsa or geriatrics - this branch is concerned with the care of the elderly. It focuses on the treatment of sickness and disease due to old age. Therapies focus on rejuvenation, longevity, memory, and strength.

Vajjikaran Chikitsa or reproductive health - this involves sexual health and treatment of reproductive problems such as infertility and the insufficiency of essential fluids.

Components of Ayurveda

Ayurveda has four components called chikitsa chatushpad, comprised of the physician, medicines, caretaker, and patient.

The physician should be alert and possess detailed practical knowledge of the subject. He should have a pure mind and body.

Medicine should be widely applicable therapeutically. Good quality and effective medicine should be used appropriately.

The caretaker should be compassionate, well trained, alert, wise, and clean.

The patient should be obedient, tolerant, and trust in the physician.

Five Elements Theory or Panchamahabhootha Theory

The five elements are building blocks of Ayurveda and are fundamentals of life of the entire universe (macrocosm) and as well as our body (microcosm). All changes in the world are the result of predominance and permutations of elements.

1. Earth- Prithvi, which is rigid.

2. Water- App, which causes fluidity.

3. Fire - Agni, which causes heat.

4. Air- Vayu, which causes mobility.

5. Ether - Akasa, which causes space/ emptiness.

Ether

We all know the very famous theory of relativity, which says space does not remain static; it either expands or contracts. Here, ether (space) is the gist of emptiness where other elements fill. Ether allows change and growth in the body. Ether contributes to the formation of the embryo by allowing growth and change in the body. The empty spaces in blood vessels, bladder, empty intestines, lungs are occupied by ether.

For example, the vitation of ether creates space and reduction in structure, resulting in tissue destruction. Parkinson's disease is a classic example of this. The cellular changes take place in the brain leading to the loss of dopamine-producing cells in the substantia nigra of the brain stem. So space occupies the place where there was cellular structure before. Similarly, in diabetes, pancreatic islet cells are destroyed in the pancreas.

Air

Ever heard of touch blindness? There's no medical term for loss of mechanical touch sensation, but touch blindness is for real. Here, air represents motion/ kinetic energy, oxygen, breath. Skin is its sensory organ, and hands are an organ of action. Disturbances with this element cause Problems with tactile perception and grasping. We all lose touch receptors as we age. Air is the driving force behind all motion that allows breathing, blood circulation, nerve impulses, thoughts to flow in our mind, joints to propel. For example, disturbances in the digestive system due to air causes excess flow - diarrhea, and when blocked, it results in constipation. In the heart, excess motion causes rapid heart rate, decreased flow leads to poor circulation, and blockage results in tissue death due to lack of oxygen.

Fire

We all have siblings or friends who are blind as bats. Visual senses and fire have an intimate relationship. Fire represents light, heat, energy, metabolism, thoughts, emotions, and the power of transformation. Disorders of visual perception are associated with fire. It helps us to digest ideas, food and digest visual impressions to identify images. Body functions like sweating, urination are a form of elimination of excess heat. Excess heat shows up through inflammation, bloodshot eyes, red rashes on the skin, intense mind, fever. Daily elimination of gas 1-2 times a day is simply a healthy digestive fire.

Water

We all hate days when we are sick, and our tastebuds go numb. Imagine being ageusia for life - that's scary!

The tongue is a sensory organ of water. It is in the form of saliva, blood, stomach, nerves, respiratory system, joints. Water is a protector and subsides pain and inflammation. Imbalance in water causes ageusia, the inability to taste. An interesting fact is that taste buds work only in the presence of water or saliva. Water protects the nerves of the brain by stabilizing the flow of neurological impulses. The overflowed water from the digestive system settles as plasma, fat, fluidic reproductive tissue. When there is increased water, it results in edema, obesity, genital secretions, menstrual flow, breast milk. Decreased water in the body results in dehydration, dry skin, and mucous membrane.

Earth

Did you know you may lose smell sensation if you are constipated? Let me explain to you how the earth element is deeply associated with our sense of smell, anosmia- loss of smell sensation. Both consumption and defecation balance the earth; too much release on earth causes diarrhea and too little causes constipation. Here, the rectum is an organ of action. Earth and smell are interlinked, so they have an impact on our ability to smell. It's also associated with strong bones, nails, and teeth. It lays the foundation for the growth and development of tissues.

This theory helps us figure out the patients and their personalities. It acts as a doorway to customize the best and most effective treatment plan.

Ayurveda and Food

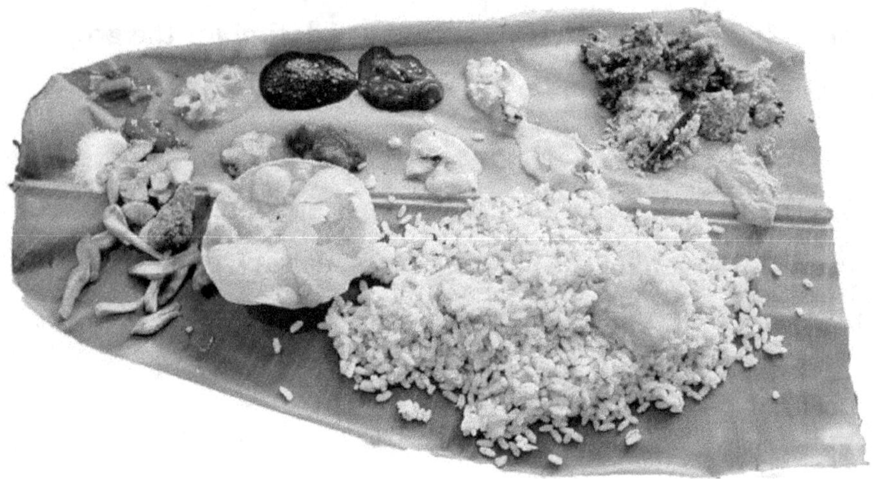

The three pillars of life are ahara - food, sleep, and celibacy. In Ayurveda, food is classified based on its taste, therapeutic properties, food compatibilities, individual's digestive ability, nature of food. Ayurveda believes in eating food based on taste (rasa). One should eat all six tastes of sweet, salty, sour, pungent, bitter, and astringent, according to Ayurveda, in each meal.

Digestion

Buffets are popular eating setups at restaurants and weddings, but the aftermath includes stomach upset, indigestion, gas, bloating, constipation. Since buffets have all kinds of food, we tend to eat without realizing food compatibility. If you are not hungry, it's because your digestive fire dint shows up. If this happens, you need to ignite your digestive fire by activating your salivary glands to produce digestive enzymes for better digestion and absorption of nutrients from food.

For proper digestion, our stomach needs suitable conditions to initiate digestion. Sit down and eat. Sitting and eating is relaxes our stomach and its ideal posture for better absorption of nutrients. Doing any kind of activities like walking, standing to inhibit digestion. I have an appetizer recipe for you to get your dodgy digestive system on track. All you need is grated ginger, a pinch of salt, few drops of lime juice to ignite that digestive fire before a meal.

Metabolism

 If you are someone who gains weight just by watching someone eat. Then your metabolism is slow as a snail, then you need to polish your metabolism. Metabolism is a process at which your body breaks down food and converts it into energy. Higher the metabolic rate, the easier for your body to shed calories and easier for you to burn fat and slim down.

Pump up your metabolism with gooseberry, Indian ginseng, licorice, nutmeg, asparagus. And herbal teas with holy basil, mint leaves, bay leaves, coriander leaves, along with two tablespoons of honey on a regular consumption basis, boosts your sluggish metabolism and helps you lose weight.

Vata Metabolism

Vatas have a fluctuating appetite. Sometimes vatas are famished and sometimes hunger-free.

Vatas are not thirsty. Vatas love eating sweet, sour, and salty foods. Vatas have weak digestion and more prone to flatulence and constipation. Vatas have sensitive defense systems and hence fall sick frequently.

Pitta Metabolism

Pittas love to eat too much and have the ability to digest quickly. Pittas are dry as dust and often feel thirsty. Pittas love bitter and sweet flavors. Pittas are good at digesting food regularly and quickly. Pittas sweat like pigs. Pittas are more prone to infections have risen in temperatures, inflammation. They have a powerful immune system.

Kapha Metabolism

Kaphas have sluggish digestion and are rarely thirsty. Kaphas should give at least three hours of time interval before consuming the next meal. They enjoy eating pungent, sweet, bitter flavors and have a powerful immune system

Wholesome and Unwholesome Foods (Pathya and Apathya)

Wholesome foods are the ones said to be nourishing all tissues of the body by restoring balance and unclogging channels, and promote health. In contrast, Unwholesome foods cause imbalance and block channels, and manifest disease. Wholesome foods and drinks are eye-pleasing, colorful, smell, and taste fresh and contribute to health. If it's wholesome for one, it might not be the same for others. They vary from person to person. Diets vary according to your body type, nature, and age. These foods are precisely suggested in disease management.

For example, iron deficiency anemia is treated with wholesome foods like Indian gooseberry, pomegranate, and buttermilk.

Curd is an unwholesome food in most doshas. Curd should not be consumed in seasons like spring, summer, and fall and during the night. Curd should be combined with green gram, sugar candy, or honey.

A patient with a cough is advised to eat vegetables, cocaine, and spices such as cardamom, long pepper, garlic, ginger, and condiments made of puffed rice. Specific taste is directly related to disease, hence better to avoid them when taking treatment for specific conditions.

Foods That are Wholesome by Nature

Red shali rice, green grams, cow milk and ghee, rainwater collected before falling on the ground, rock salt, ginger, grapes, Jivanti leaves (Leptadenia reticulata), and sesame oil.

Foods That are Unwholesome by Nature

Yawak among paddy, safflower oil, black gram, sheep milk and ghee, beef meat, mustard leaf, potato, monkey fruit

Best Dietary Habits According to Ayurveda

Eat lots of fruits and vegetables because they are natural cleansers for the body.

Eat bioavailable foods. Now bioavailable foods are eating your veggies cooked instead of eating them raw. Raw veggies may contain more vitamins and nutrients but are hard on our digestive system.

Start your day with lukewarm water. This ancient ayurvedic practice has been gaining popularity lately to aid in weight loss. By increasing your body's temperature, metabolism increases, helping us lose weight.

Sit and sip water. Sit down and have water that's at room temperature. Don't drink too much water before or after a meal. The rule of thumb is your stomach should be filled with 50% food, 25% water, and 25% should be left empty for space.

Eat three hours before bedtime. When at sleep, the body repairs, heals and restores. If the body is diverted into the digestive process is ceased. So, the last meal should be light and three hours before sleep.

Drink herbal tea every day. Herbal teas calm your mind. Chamomile tea helps People suffering from Insomnia. It is rich in antioxidants lowering the risk of diseases related to heart and cancer. Chamomile tea helps to put us to sleep. Vatas can be calmed by warm spicy herbal teas of cinnamon, cloves, and ginger. Pittas can be calmed with herbs that have cooling effects, such as peppermint, coriander, and rose. Kaphas can increase their energy and digestion with black pepper, licorice, and cardamom.

Steps to Ayurvedic Eating

Eating in this age of dieting, in a world of social media influencers constantly influencing us, no wonder why we are obsessed with fancy fad diets. Diets like Keto, general motors diet, vegan-diet, Atkins diet paleo-diet are tempting but are unsustainable and come with a heavy price and side effects in the long run. Unlike modern diet plans, Ayurveda personalizes diet plans about foods you should be eating and avoiding based on your body type, and you will learn about how to cook and staple foods and recipes in further coming chapters.

5 Must-Haves in Ayurvedic Eating

1. Ghee – the clarified butter is a staple and most rejuvenating food in Ayurveda; it helps in digestion and is an excellent transporting medium for the body to utilize nutrients.

2. Turmeric - This golden spice that every Indian swears by is used for the past 4000 years; it has a plethora of benefits. Curcumin, an antioxidant in turmeric lately turmeric is sold in the form of chewing tablets for oral cancer, liver problems.

3. Fenugreek seeds - Although, fenugreek is not so common in the western kitchen. These bitter-tasting tiny seeds are stress relievers. Teas made with fenugreek seeds, cinnamon, honey, lemon juice, and holy basil or simply soaking them overnight and consuming in the morning helps too.

4. Ginger - this powerful root is popular among people with digestive problems like nausea, bloating, and indigestion. It has a unique ability to gently initiate peristalsis, helping food move through the gastrointestinal tract. It also has anti-inflammatory properties.

5. Jaggery - this superfood sweetener is rich in vitamin B, calcium, copper, zinc, and phosphorus. Finish your lunch with little jaggery and ghee. This powerful combo is rich in iron and essential fatty acids. It not only keeps your sweet tooth at bay but also helps with hormones and immunity.

Benefits of Ayurvedic Eating

One can benefit from ayurvedic eating because it encourages us to eat whole foods packed with nutrients and fiber instead of refined foods. Refined foods are stripped off from nutrients and lack fiber. Boosts weight loss, too.

Ayurveda promotes mindfulness and helps to stick to new and healthy behaviors.

People practicing Ayurveda and yoga had improved psychosocial health; it helps one by cleansing and detoxification.

Ayurvedic diets reduce plaque buildup and cholesterol and fats in arteries. Further reducing cardiovascular risk and blood pressure.

Ayurvedic diets reduce inflammation.

An Ayurvedic diet is greatly known for keeping cancer at bay.

Ayurvedic diets increase vitality, pump energy, and make you feel light by decreased lethargy and mood swings. Ayurveda has been sought as a popular therapy for stress management and anxiety issues.

Tips for Good Digestion

Allow 3 hours for food to digest. Let the true hunger return before consuming another meal, or it leads to poor digestion. Do not overeat and avoid eating straight after a full meal. You are likely to end up feeling heavy, bloated, and lethargic if not done so. In general, waiting for 3 hours between meals is a good idea. Kaphas should wait longer since they have a slower digestive system.

Sit down while you eat your meals. Eating in a sitting down posture is ideal for smooth digestion; it also keeps gastric problems at bay. Our stomach is in a relaxed posture, and our awareness is of the taste, texture, and smell of the food; it will greatly improve digestion.

Pair your foods wisely. According to Ayurveda, some food combinations don't go well on your stomach. They disturb the normal functioning of gastric fire and upset your stomach, causing Indigestion, gas formation. Some incompatible combinations are milk and banana, honey and ghee. Yoghurt with sour fruits, eggs, and milk.

Your lunch should be the largest meal you eat in a day. Digestive fire is strongest when the sun is strongest, that is, between 12 and 2 pm. Ideally, lunch should be the large meal and dinner, the lighter, the better.

Drink lassi during lunchtime. Lassi is nothing but sweetened yoghurt. Add sugar and water into plain yoghurt. Blend it for a minute. Lassi is an excellent source of probiotics, contains good bacteria called lactobacilli that lubricates our intestines and help digestion go smoothly. Lassi also helps in reducing gas, bloating, and boosts metabolism, in turn, helps lose weight.

Foods to Incorporate or Avoid for Different Doshas

Foods Vatas Should Eat

Proteins like eggs, seafood like fish and shrimp, tofu, dairy products like milk, ghee, butter, cheese. Fruits like bananas, cherries, apricots, strawberries, avocados, peaches, blueberries, mangoes, grapefruits, plums, figs, cherries, melons, oranges, nectarines. Veggies like onions, green beans, celeriac, leafy green vegetables, radishes, peas, sweet potatoes, turnips, celery, carrots, beets. Consume them cooked instead of raw. Legumes like lentils, chickpeas, mung beans. Grains like cooked rice, semolina, oats, spelts, wheat. Nuts like walnuts, pistachios, almonds. Seeds like sunflower and flax seeds. Herbs like basil, thyme, oregano. Spices like black pepper, cardamom, ginger, cloves, cumin.

Foods Vatas Should Avoid

Proteins like red meat, fruits like unripened and dried pears, raisins, pomegranates, cranberries. Avoid raw Vegetables and cooked cabbage, broccoli, cauliflower, mushrooms, tomatoes, potatoes. Legumes like beans, such as kidney beans, navy beans, and black beans. Grains like barley, corn, rye, wheat, quinoa, buckwheat, millets. Herbs and spices that taste bitter like parsley, thyme, coriander.

Foods Pittas Should Consume

Protein sources like egg whites, tofu, dairy products like milk, butter, and ghee. Fruits like apples, oranges, pineapples, pears, damsons, avocados, raisins, mangoes, and melons. Eat them when fully ripe and sweet. Vegetables like cauliflower, leafy greens, cucumber, cabbage, cauliflower, celery, zucchini, chard, squash, carrots, broccoli, brussels sprouts, mushrooms, green peppers, lettuce, asparagus, and celery.

Legumes like lentils, chickpeas, and beans like mung beans, lima beans, black beans, kidney beans. Grains like oats, wheat, brown rice, barley. Nuts and seeds like coconut, flax seeds, chia seeds, sunflower, and pumpkin seeds. Herbs like cilantro, dill. Spices like black pepper, turmeric, cumin, cinnamon.

Foods Pittas Should Avoid

Proteins like egg yolks, red meat, seafood. Dairy like buttermilk, cheese, sour cream. Fruits like grapes, papaya,

apricots, sour cherries, fruits that are sour and unripe.
Vegetables like beets, onions, chili peppers, eggplant,
tomatoes. Grains like rye, millets, brown rice, corn. Nuts like
almonds, pine nuts, walnuts, cashews, pistachios. Seeds like
sesame seeds. Avoid spices that are not mentioned above.

Foods Kaphas Should Consume

For protein, consume seafood and egg whites. Dairy like goat
milk, skim milk, soy milk. Fruits like pears, raisins, apricots,
apples, mangos, berries like cranberries, blueberries,
cherries, pomegranates. Vegetables like artichokes, onions,
asparagus, broccoli, potatoes, beetroot, eggplant, ladies
finger, chicory, lettuce, mushrooms, fennel, garlic, celeriac,
spinach, radish. Dried fruits like figs, prunes, and raisins.
Legumes like chickpeas, navy beans, black beans, lentils.
Grains like rye, quinoa, barley, corn, all types of millets,
buckwheat, oats, couscous. Herbs like thyme, basil, oregano.
Spices like cinnamon, cumin, turmeric, ginger, and black
pepper. Seeds like sunflower seeds, pumpkin seeds, flax
seeds.

Foods Kaphas Should Avoid

Proteins like egg yolks, red meat, shrimp. Fruits like

bananas, fresh figs, coconut, mangoes. Vegetables like cucumbers, sweet potatoes, zucchini. Legumes like miso, soybeans, kidney beans. Grains like cereal, rice, wheat. Nuts and seeds like cashews, brazil nuts, pecans, walnuts, pine nuts, sesame seeds.

Eat According to Your Dosha

Vatas favor consuming warm, nourishing foods that are fairly heavy in texture.

Warm milk, soups, stews, broths, hot cereals, and freshly baked bread, cream and butter, nut butter, raw nuts are great for vatas. Foods that have flavors of salty, sour, and sweet, along with soothing foods, are great options to look for. Adding butter and good fats can help you with balancing vata. Look for Fruits that are well ripened. Make Warming herbal teas part of your daily routine. Herbal teas that have spices like fresh ginger root, cinnamon, cardamom. Savoring Hot ginger tea every day is a great support to vatas. Avoid caffeinated drinks and candies, cold beverages, salads and raw veggies, unripe fruits, as they are astringent.

Pittas can favor by both cool and warm foods with fairly heavy texture. Flavors like bitter, astringent, sweet are ideal for you. Consume foods like salads with lemon juice, milk, grains, vegetables as much as you can, and ice creams on hot days. Herbal teas with licorice root, mint pacify pitta. Cinnamon toast, chilled cereal, and apple tea for breakfast is a good choice. Vegetarian foods are best for pittas. Avoid hot steaming foods, fermented foods, cheese, honey, egg yolks, coffee, nuts, hot drinks, oily foods, butter, sour cream, vinegar, pickles, and red meat as they tend to heat the body.

Kaphas favor warm, dry, light meals. Raw vegetables and fruits work best for kaphas. Any spicy food is good for Kaphas. Indian and Mexican cuisine suit best, especially, dishes that are hot and spicy is good during winters. Cooking methods that are dry like grilling, broiling, baking, sautéing over moist cooking methods such as steaming, poaching, boiling. To stimulate appetite kaphas need to eat romaine lettuce, tonic water, endive, and spices like fenugreek, turmeric, cumin, sesame seed. Kaphas should watch their salt intake to avoid fluid retention and reduce their sugar and fats intake. Avoid deep-fried foods, dairy products. Keep your lunch large and dinner small.

What is Digestive Fire?

The idea of digestive fire is a concept based on the functions of the stomach, its strength, amount of stomach acids, bile in the gastrointestinal tract, digestive enzymes. The teamwork of these juices helps to dissolve the food we ate into essential building blocks for strength and energy, nutrition. Digestive fire, or agni, is a metaphor for the digestive system. Agni's functions include sense perception such as touch, taste, vitality, hearing, appetite, clarity, combustion, alertness, and metabolic functions absorption, digestion, and mental assimilation. Our bellies have the fire to digest food and control brain centers, and nourish them with its vapors by releasing nerve impulses that in turn secrete hormones and release enzymes. Signs of balance in agni are emotions like intelligence, courage, lucid. Signs of imbalance are anger, fear, and confusion occur.

What is Ama?

Ama is toxins within the body due to an improper diet, undigested and unabsorbed, and is fertile ground for breeding diseases. Ama clogs all channels and causes stagnation of nutrients from reaching cells and wastes from excretion. For example, kidney failure is caused due to accumulation of urea. Urea has to be eliminated from the body. So, here urea is ama. The interesting thing is that the concept of free radicals in modern medicine is taken from

Ayurveda - the concept of ama.

Ama is a forerunner of illness. Ama has germs, undigested food, the bad cholesterol. Ama is formed by bad eating habits, stress, and incompatible foods.

Symptoms of ama include disturbances in excretory functions, heaviness, indigestion, excess salivation and anorexia, white coating on the tongue, and loss of taste sensation.

Treat ama with herbs and spices such as guduchi (Tinospora cordifolia), ginger, neem, castor, turmeric. These work best for treating ama. Alongside taking herbs, the first and foremost treatment is fasting. It ignites the digestive fire. Second-line treatment includes the application of heat with sand in cloth bags as it causes sweating and relieves pain and swelling called dry sudation therapy. Panchakarma is also advised.

What is Ojas?

Oja is a liquid in the body that's the essence of all body parts and concerned with preventing disease and promoting overall health. Charaka described it as a yellowish, white, red liquid that dwells in the heart in oja of the body.

Let's say someone is suffering from a cold and is on medication; oja is the one that is responsible for metabolizing medicine and targets the organ that needs to be treated and promotes healing. A person with a good amount of oja has good immunity and falls sick less frequently from cold, cough, and fever.

Consuming ghee, milk, and practicing ayurvedic eating yoga and pranayama will increase oja.

Achieving Balance and Working Out

How Vatas Can Achieve Balance

Stick to the foods and dietary guidelines mentioned above. Stay calm and in a comforting environment. Go for ayurvedic massage sessions as they are soothing and grounding for Vatas. Avoid breezy and dry climates. Travel less and avoid noisy, crowded places and talk less. Keep yourself warm and sleep tight.

Workouts for Vatas

Vatas have smaller body frame, weak digestive system, and are underweight. You have a hard time gaining weight and must focus on building stronger bones and muscles. Vatas are naturally energetic; they enjoy doing fast-paced workouts like dancing, cardio, running, yoga, walking is good for vatas. Lunges, squats, resistance training, and low-intensity exercises, and yoga are excellent options for you.

How Pittas Can Achieve Balance

Alongside following dietary guidelines mentioned above, practice meditating and aromatherapy with cooling scents such as lavender, sandalwood, rose, and mint that smell heavenly; massages are a great help too.

Making your visit to a good spa once in a while is a great idea to relax. You have powerful stamina and average stature. You are athletic by nature and love exercising to push yourself. Do not workout in hot, humid places. Workout during cooler times, in the fresh air, and hydrate yourself. Be patient and considerate towards others. Engage in thoughtful sessions and avoid situations of disputes.

Workouts for Pittas

Pittas are hot by nature and have warm bodies. To counterbalance your energy, you should do non-competitive, low intensity, and relaxing workouts. The medium pace and moderate-intensity Workouts will do. Yin yoga, pilates, trampolining, and walking are some best choices you can make. Swimming is best for your hot body.

How Kaphas Can Achieve Balance

Stick to the dietary guidelines in the diet above. Be an early raiser and sleepless. Avoid catnaps during day time. Allow yourself to adapt to new changes, challenges, and adventures in life. Escape from stagnation and being lethargic. Meditation and pranayama (breathing exercises) can make a lot of difference.

Workouts for Kaphas

Kapha types have bigger frames, great physical strength, exercising regularly is extremely important to curb that excess Kapha energy. It is difficult to exercise when you are feeling low, but it is crucial to activating your body and mind. You should try fast-paced exercises, due to high endurance you can perform exercises for a longer period. Exercises like cardio, Tabata, HIIT, plyometrics, Zumba dance, or simply jogging are great. Eat light and healthy. Group activity is a great option as it keeps you motivated.

Do's and Don'ts of Ayurveda

Do's of Ayurveda

Eat foods that are healthy and compatible.

Bathe twice daily.

Shave and cut your hair and nails thrice a fortnight.

Maintain hygiene in body openings and keep your feet clean.

Wear clean clothes.

Eat according to your body constitution.

Go to bed early.

Exercise regularly.

Wake up to Brahma muhurta, one and a half hours before sunrise; it is the best time to meditate.

Don'ts of Ayurveda

Avoid suppressing natural body urges like urination, sneezing, yawning, hiccups, coughing, hunger, farting, stools, thirst, sleep.

Don't apply face packs during the night.

Don't overindulge in celibacy.

Don't eat food of similar tastes every day.

Avoid excessive use of sense organs like your eyes by playing on phones.

Avoid people with negative emotions.

Avoid sleeping late at night.

Talk softly, don't be loud.

What the Ayurvedic Lifestyle Can Heal

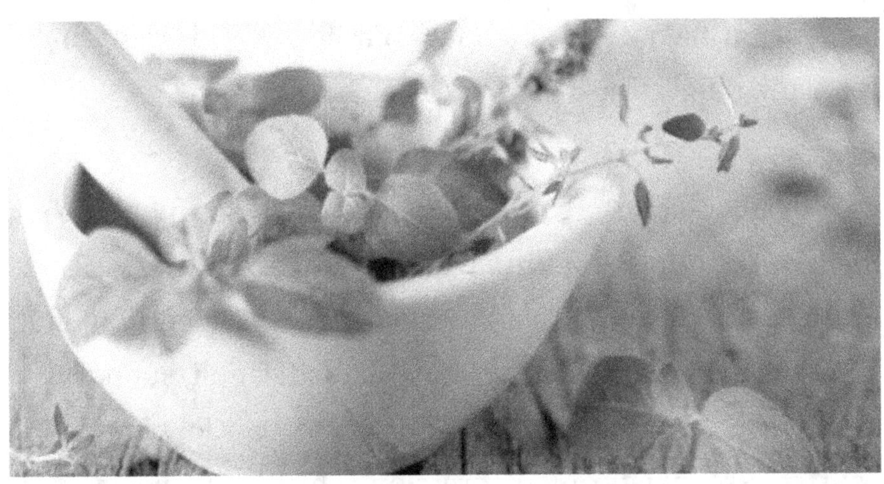

As we learned, Ayurveda is a way of living and preventing rather than healing. Now the real question is, does Ayurveda help in sickness? The answer is yes!

There are two kinds of ailments, one is infectious, and the other is chronic. Infectious ailments act through external invasion into the body. Here, you must go see a doctor, and it has to be dealt with through medicine. In such cases, Ayurveda or meditation won't probably save you.

But a chronic ailment is when our body is creating the

problem and causing disease. But why would our own body turn against us when every cell in the body is programmed for positive health? The answer is, you are not keeping those cells and your body happy and not doing things that need to be done for them to function for your health. This imbalance is creating illness instead of creating health.

70% of all ailments are self-created, and we must not lay the blame on our bodies. Chronic problems like diabetes, hormonal imbalance, cardiovascular diseases, digestion and bloating, insomnia, inflammation, detoxification, subpar immunity, skin problems, blood pressure, hair loss, weight gain, stress, anxiety, and depression, which, are longstanding and require lifestyle changes like specific ayurvedic diet for each problem, yoga, and meditation. One can adapt to Ayurveda as a complementary medicine and heal from chronic ailments through ayurvedic methods.

Anxiety, Stress, and Depression

It is quite normal to feel anxious about taking SATs, moving to a new city, or investing in stocks. But when this anxious feeling stays with you all the time, then it's a matter of concern. If you have ever felt anxious about passing a day, entering an elevator, leaving your house, or doing things that you would normally enjoy doing, then this anxiety disorder must be treated before it's too late. As per the American psychiatric association, 6.8 million adults suffer from anxiety every year, and its prevalence in women is twice as much as in men.

Anxiety is an emotional state of being tense, worried thoughts, and increased blood pressure. Physical symptoms include rapid heartbeat, sweating, dizziness, trembling.

Types of anxiety disorders include:

> A Panic disorder is when you experience panic attacks that recur unusually, and the fear of the next pain attack bothers you all the time.

> Phobias include fear of a place, a thing, or an activity.

> A Separation disorder is where you fear being away from your home or pet, loved ones. Usually, boarding schools can give this anxiety disorder in kids.

> Social anxiety disorder is the fear of being judged by others during social gatherings, such as stage fear.

Post-traumatic stress is anxiety after a traumatic event and its haunting memories. Examples include domestic violence, sexual abuse.

Obsessive-compulsive disorder is having irrational, obsessive thoughts, compulsions to perform things in a certain way, and repeated behavior.

Illness anxiety disorder is feeling anxious about health.

Depression

Depression is real, and it is beyond sadness. But it is the most underrated stigma around. It is leading to hindrance from getting treated. It is estimated that 17.3 million adults, that is 7.15% of adults in America had an experience of a major depressive episode at least once in their lifetimes. And its prevalence is higher among females. Depression is not a myth, and famous people like Robin Williams, Kate Spade, Avicii, and Chester Bennington wouldn't commit suicide owing to depression if it was just a normal illness. Symptoms include lack of interest in daily activities, insomnia or hypersomnia, weight gain or loss, feeling worthless, guilt, lack of attention, suicidal thoughts, and thinking about death. Seek help before you turn into a full-on depressive mania.

The science behind depression is an imbalance in neurotransmitters like dopamine, norepinephrine, and serotonin that have an impact on mood regulation.

Stress

Stress is our body's reaction to a possibly harmful situation. To fight stress, the brain triggers our fight or flight response. When under stress, chemicals and hormones like adrenaline and cortisol flood the body, known as the adrenalin rush. Stress can lead to high blood pressure, damaged blood vessels, heart attack, stroke, headaches, insomnia, and weight gain.

How to Deal with Anxiety and Depression Using Ayurveda

Meditation

Meditation is focusing our mind on one thought, and only that one thought, to achieve clear thinking and emotional calmness and to stay stable. When we meditate, we instill deep sighted benefits in our lives that could go a long way.

1. Get comfy and stay put for a couple of minutes and just focus on deep breathing.

2. Try to feel your breath, be it in your belly or nose. Pay attention to your breath while you inhale and exhale.

3. Continue to follow your breath for two minutes by deeply inhaling, expanding your belly, and then slowly exhale, extending your breath out, contracting your belly.

Lifestyle and Dietary Changes

Eat foods that are mentioned in foods to balance vata dosha. Dietary foods that are rich in selenium, magnesium, zinc, omega 3 fatty acids, probiotics, vitamin D, flavonoids, antioxidants, and foods that have anti-inflammatory properties work best for mental health disorders.

Selenium deficiency leads to mood disorders like depression, and reports on supplementation of selenium to improve mood have positive results.

The major food sources of selenium in the Western diet are

seafood, bread, macaroni, organ meat, grains, liver, poultry and eggs, cottage cheese, and yogurt. Vegetables like carrots, garlic, potatoes, spinach, green peas, lentils, lettuce. Brazil nuts are a gift from the amazon forest, as they have extremely high amounts of selenium in them. one brazil nut has 96mcg. Whereas 400mcg/day is the maximum value for an adult.

Fatty fish offer high amounts of Omega 3 fatty acids. Zinc from red meat, oysters, crab; magnesium from green leafy veggies.

Lifestyle changes like yoga, meditation, mantra meditation, and engaging in your favorite hobby can be of great help.

Ayurvedic Herbs

Ashwagandha or Withania somnifera is a prominent herb in Ayurveda, which can be used as a stress buster, and energy booster. It also helps in improving one's concentration. For over 3000 years in India, the people over there are benefitting from the adaptogens in it, which have a significantly positive effect on hormones in regulating stress. It reduces cortisol levels and aids in better sleep.

Chamomile has been used by the ancient Greeks and Romans for its calming effects. It is well known for inducing sleep and its use in generalized anxiety disorder treatment. It has phenolic, that is known for relaxing our brain.

Lavender, the aromatic herb that's known for its sedative effect on brain centers that are related to emotions, thereby reducing stress and anxiety. It also reduces cortisol levels (stress hormone).

Passionflower has flavonoids and alkaloids that relieve anxiety-induced insomnia. It's a potentially underrated herb that helps insomniacs. It reduces anticipatory fear by relaxing the brain.

Kava is a potent herb and the best-researched herb for anxiety. It takes 15-20 minutes for its effects to kick in, making it an instantaneous anxiety-reliever during flight and fright response in situations like near accidents. Kava should be used as an emergency remedy only due to its damaging effects on the liver.

Ayurvedic Tools to Deal With Stress, Anxiety, and Depression

The below-mentioned tools will calm your mind, restoring balance in mind, spirit, and body. They will enhance physical energy, mental clarity, and relax your mind. Ancient Ayurvedic bathing rituals were considered to be highly effective therapeutic activities that included luxurious full-body warm oil massage with herbal oils followed by application of sandalwood paste, floral waters, and aromatherapy with essential oils.

Calming effects of Certain fragrances help you relax and ease up. Put three drops of basil oil, clove oil, frankincense, orange into a diffuser or in water for a hot bath. Bathing with turmeric, milk, rose petals, and honey was an ancient ayurvedic way of bathing.

Abhyanga is an Ayurvedic daily self-massage of the head, hands and feet. Massaging your scalp with sesame oil or rich coconut oil and continue on to the forehead and temples for 3 minutes every day. This improves blood circulation and relaxes our mind. Oga and breathing sessions followed by meditation and chanting mantras like OMKAR or Gayatri Mantra once or twice a day is beneficial.

Nadi shodhana, aka alternate nostril breathing, is a practice of rhythmically and knowingly changing the flow of air from one nostril to another known as pranayama; it is known to soothe our nervous system and relieve anxiety. Other activities like walking in the forest or your lawn alongside water bodies will enhance the mood.

The below-mentioned therapies are general stress management therapy procedures. You can ask for these treatments on your visit to any ayurvedic center.

Abyanga: Full body massage with the use of medicated herbal oils that lasts 60 minutes to relieve tensions from joints and muscles.

Pizchil: Head massage that lasts 15 minutes and oil pouring and massage to deep tissues to strengthen hormonal secretions.

Sirodhara: Flow of herbal oils, milk or buttermilk onto the forehead and head massage for 45 minutes to calm your nervous system.

Sirovasthi: Placing a cup on your head with lukewarm herbal oils in it for 45 minutes to calm your brain and nervous system.

Talam: Application of herbal powder mixed with medicated oil on top of the head.

Talapothichil: Applying herbal pastes on to the body. Followed by a steam bath.

Ayurveda & Yoga - a Potent Recipe to Handle Depression and Anxiety

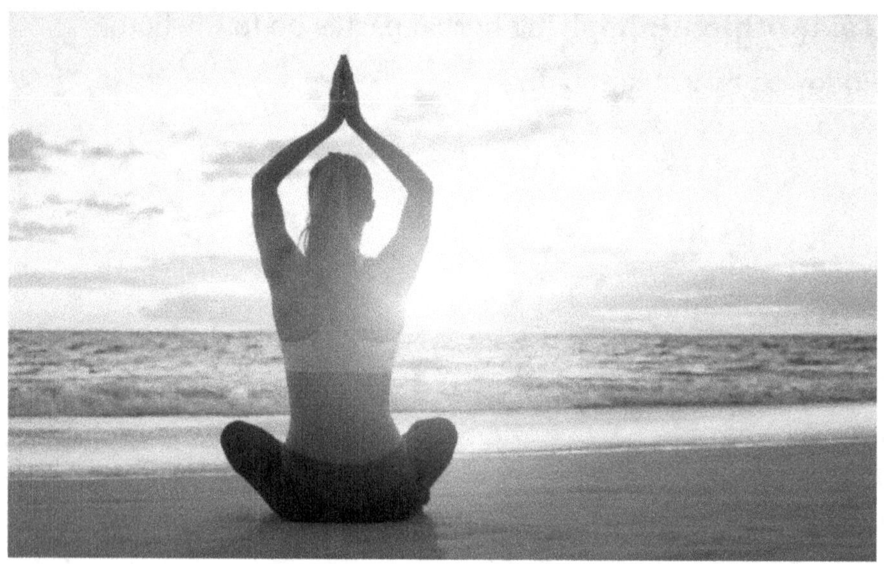

Although yoga and Ayurveda are two different sciences, they share the same Vedic roots. Yoga is a sister science of Ayurveda and springs from the same Vedic system as Ayurveda. They follow the same principles and believes that drive us to holistic wellbeing.

While yoga treats with balancing the mind, body, and soul, Ayurveda treats with the physical and mental wellbeing through lifestyle changes and ayurvedic diet. Yoga's ability to combat physical and mental problems is a good reason to try it out.

Researchers from Harvard have interesting things to say, that even at this initial phase of research, basic yoga practice at regular intervals seems to be interlinked with increased wellbeing and better sleep, mindfulness, and weight loss, along with boosting emotions like compassion and gratitude. Through its stressbusting effects, yoga also has an impact on a cellular level and slows down the aging process.

Yoga can improve multiple things in our life, all at once. Yoga generates positive feedback loops that further promote healthy habits.

Must-Do Asanas for Complete Well-Being

Mountain pose: Tadasana

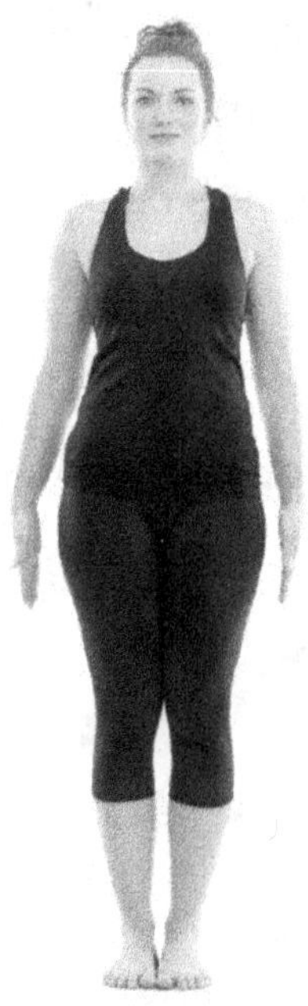

Maintain this posture for 10 breaths. You can do the 'namaste' position by bringing the palms together in front of your chest. It generates a sense of stability and prepares you for the rest of the session.

Boat pose: Naukasana

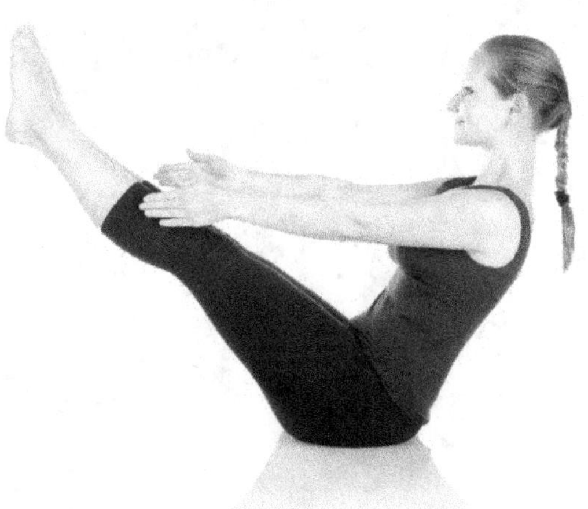

This asana is excellent for ab-strengthening. Breathe in and out, use your core muscles as you exhale to lift your hands, legs, and torso. Look at your toes and hold this pose for five breaths. It also helps strengthens the abdominal muscles and improves digestion.

Warrior pose: Virabhadrasana

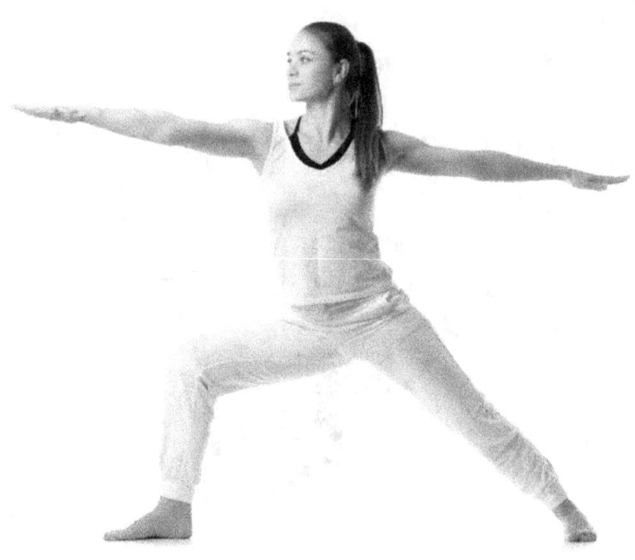

Legs should be three feet apart and hands in the line of the shoulder. Look ahead at your fingertips. Hold this pose for five breaths. It boosts self-confidence and stamina. It also corrects flat feet.

Powerful pose: Utkatasana

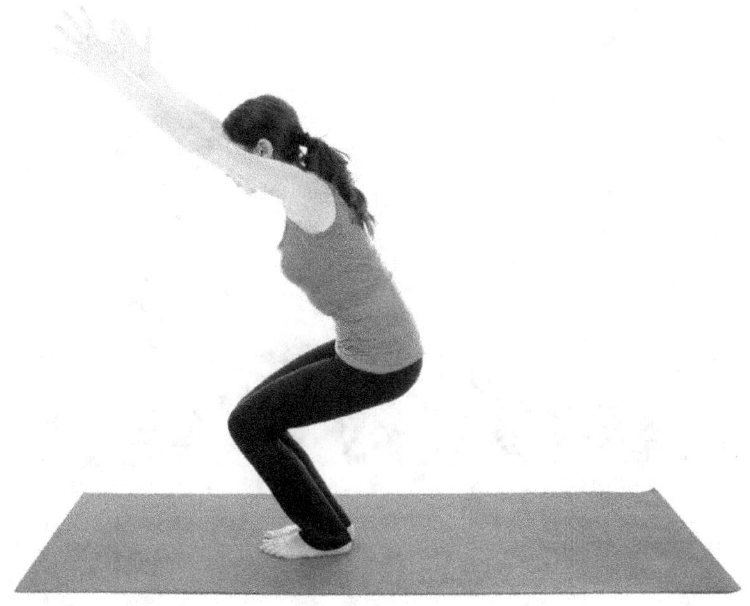

Begin in the mountain pose. As you breathe in, take your hands up from the sides and touch both above your head, stretch your torso, and elongate the spine. Now, keeping the feet firmly grounded, breathe out and bend your knees and go as low as you can. Hold this pose for good five breaths. This pose helps you to stay focused and balanced. It strengthens calves and thighs.

Cobra pose: Bhujangasana

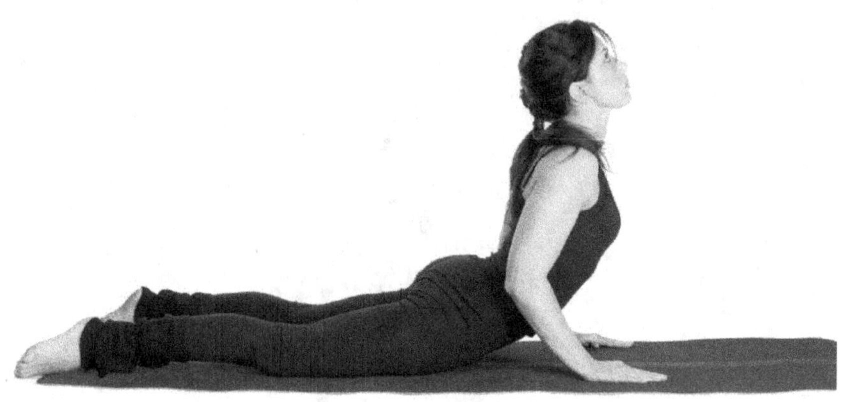

Start by keeping your forehead on the mat and inhale. Then, lift your head and shoulders higher, and slide your hands forward. Hold this position for five breaths and relax. This enhances the backbend curve and spinal flexibility. It also reduces stiff neck and back, relieves sciatica pain, and firm glutes.

Mind, Body, and Consciousness

The Western world has always seen the mind, body, and consciousness as three different things. However, that's not the case in the eastern part of the world. What I'm saying is, even though they are three different things, they're ultimately connected to each other and work in a rhythmic flow.

Ever wondered how you feel cluttered and confused in your mind when you're all worked up in your night shift?! Well, when your body is tired, so does your mind, and vice versa. Anyhow, I'd like to help you with keeping all things healthy, so that you, as a whole person, stay happy and healthy. And how are you going to do that?! Yoga, my dear friends!

These Yoga Asanas will relieve your stress and give you peace of mind.

Bow pose: Dhanurasana

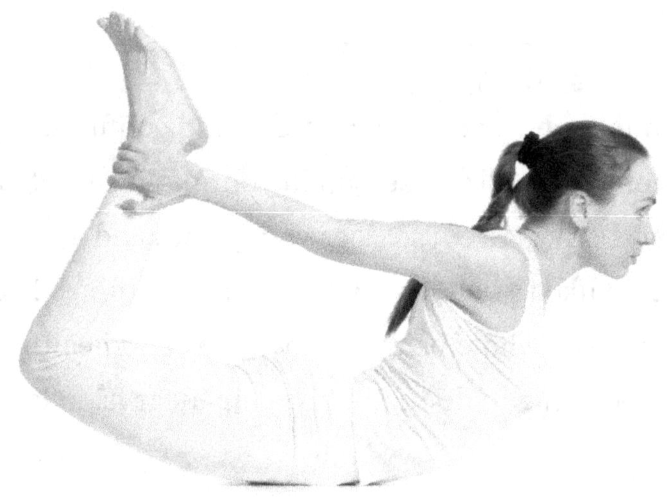

A famous yoga asana, which is not only simple but also super-beneficial. People with spinal cord problems can be greatly benefited from this. But, keep in mind, if you have any stomach-related issues, consult your doctor before performing this asana.

Fish pose: Matsyasana

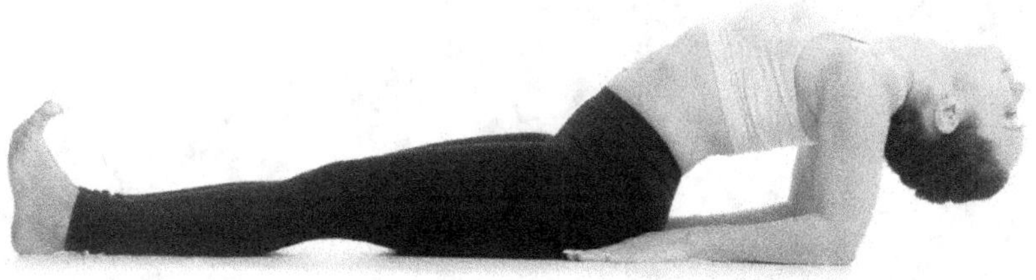

Matsya literally translates to fish in Sanskrit. Here, you bend your back in such a way, your spinal cord gets finally free from all the stiffness you've been accumulating. It helps you strengthen your upper back and upper neck muscles. People suffering from depression and anxiety could get serious help by working on their upper neck muscles.

One-legged forward bend: Janu Shirsasana

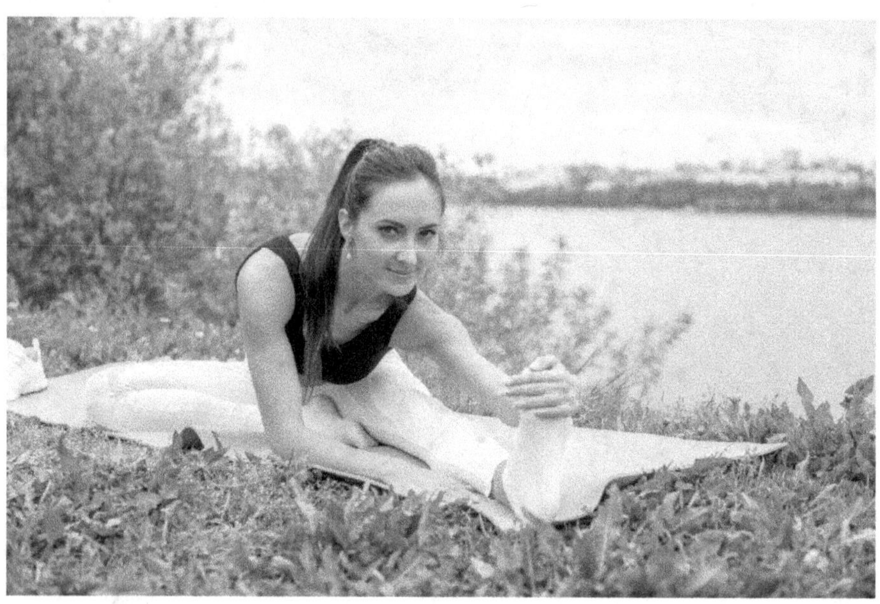

This pose helps you stretch and strengthen your inguinal region, vertebral column, shoulders, and hamstring as well. I would say this is one of those yoga asanas, which helps you work on multiple parts of your body at the same time.

Bridge pose: Setubandhasana

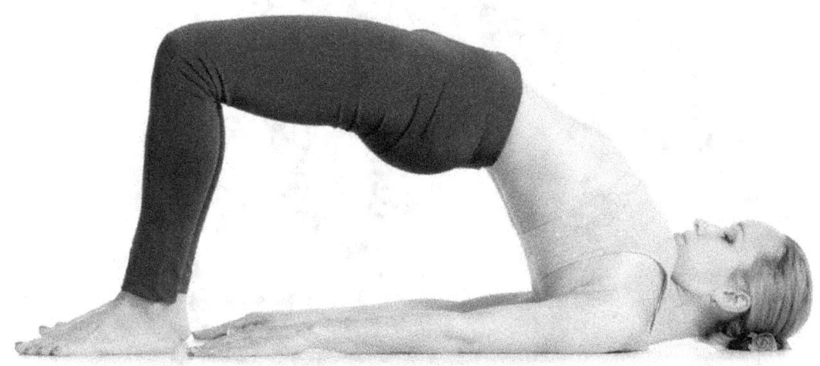

It is also known as sarvangasana. In Sanskrit, sarvanga translates to "all body parts." It might seem very basic on the first look, however, don't underestimate the power of this yoga pose. Not only does it help you work on your whole body, it mainly emphasizes on strengthening your thorax, neck, and vertebral column. Do you know what it means? Well, the muscles in these parts, when properly taken care of, help you find relief from anxiety, depression, and other mental health issues.

Cat stretch: Marjariasana

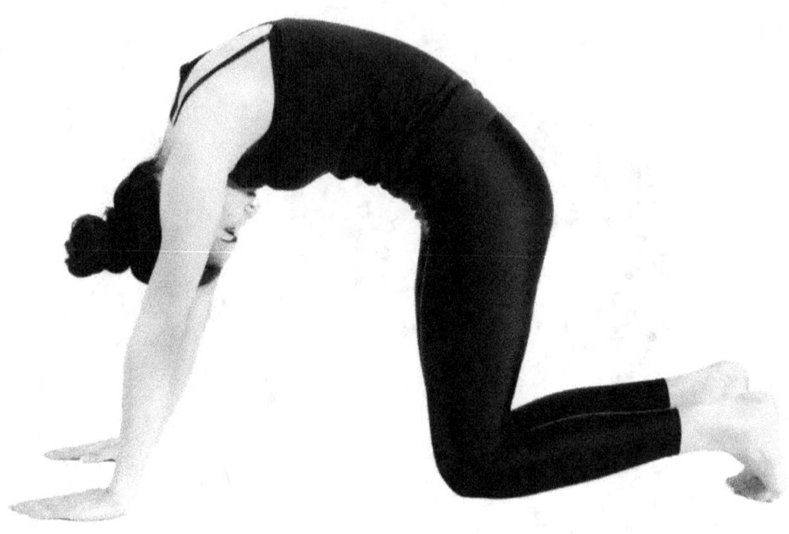

Yep! You're going to look like a cat while doing this pose, and you shouldn't be embarrassed by that. Why?! Well, this yoga asana is such an awesome and helpful thing, if done properly, helps you deal with torso-related issues, which is quite an important thing.

Two-legged forward bend: Paschimottanasana

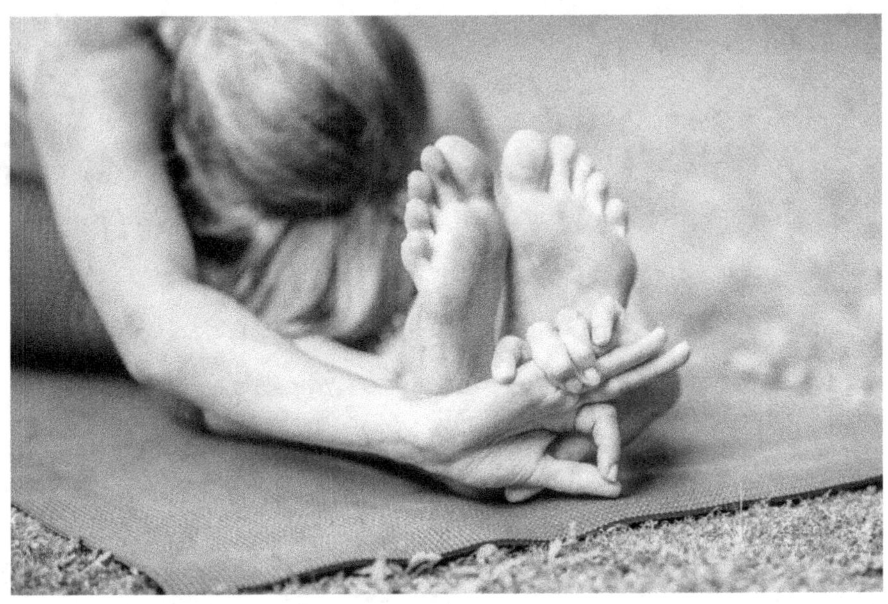

If you're an aspiring athlete, you can't afford missing this Yoga pose. It helps you work on complicated muscle streams in areas like vertebral column, hamstring, and shoulder, all at the same time. Here, you'll be performing an intense dorsal stretch, which helps you relieve all the fitness related issues.

Downward facing dog: Adhomukha Shwanasana

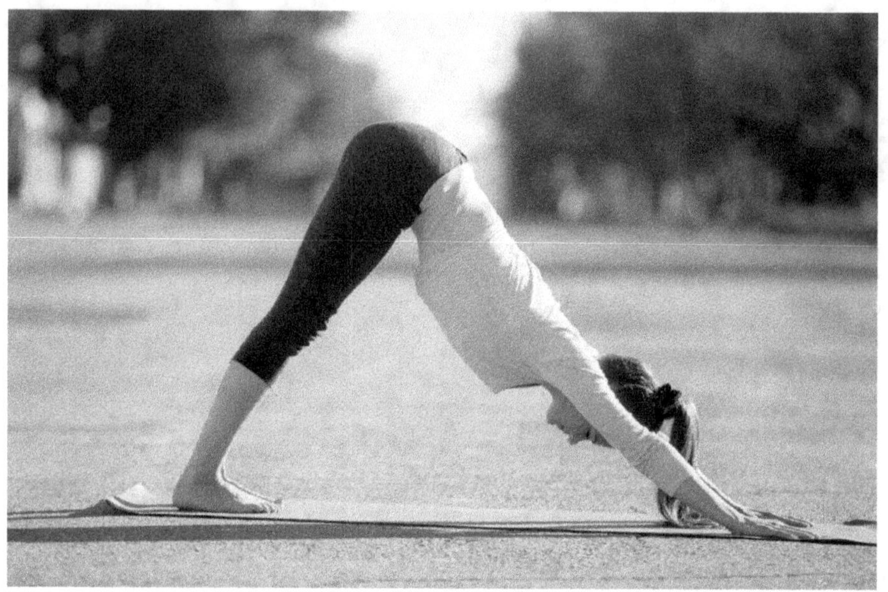

This is usually performed after other significant Yoga poses such as surya namaskara. However, you can also solely proceed with as well. It helps you stretch and work on all the core muscles in your arms and legs.

Headstand : Shirshasana

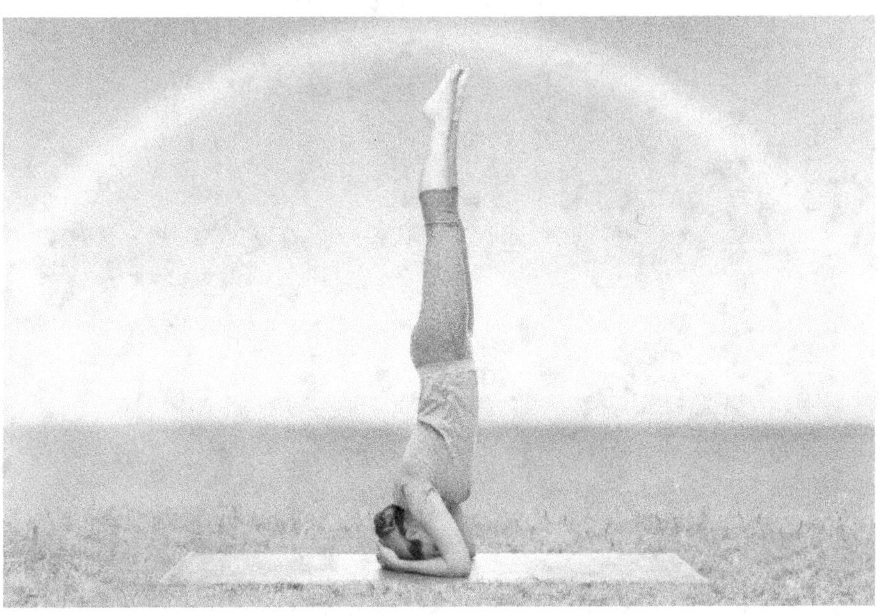

From my personal experience, this is the best yoga pose to relieve you from anxiety. But, there's a catch, while doing this pose, in the initial days, I felt dizziness. However, after persistently sticking with it, I've started feeling better and better. Make sure that you're focused while doing this, as it's quite difficult to master staying in balance while performing this asana.

Corpse pose: Shavasana

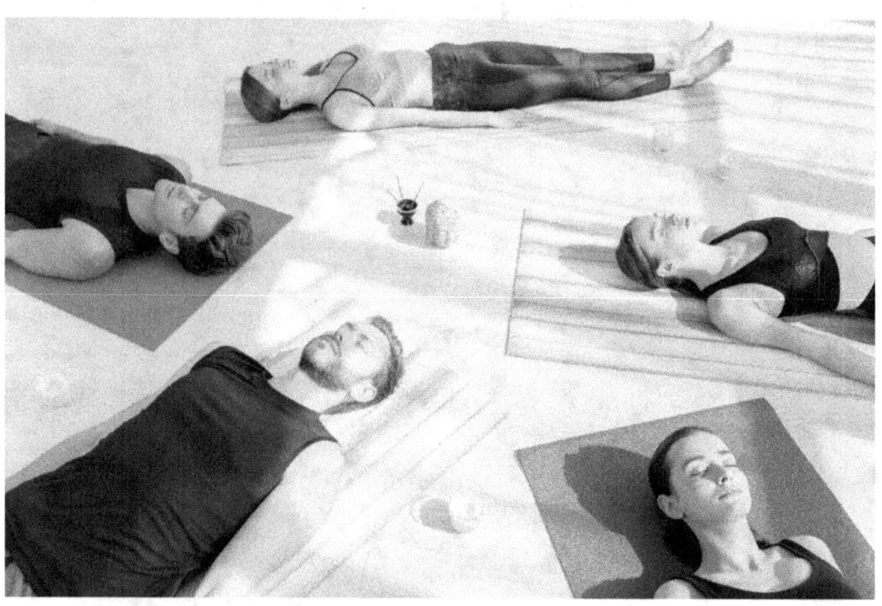

Just lay down, like a corpse. No, seriously! As simple and weird as it may sound, this is one of the most popular, effective, and easy yoga poses. It helps you relax your body and mind, letting you ease down, and get rid of all the stress, whether it is physical or psychological.

Seasonal Yoga Practices

As far as I know, there's no other medical system that comes close to Ayurveda, when stressing about the importance of seasonal health practices. In Sanskrit, it's called ritu charya -

ritu meaning season/time, and charya meaning regime. This system helps us balance and maintain our health, following unique methods for different seasons. No more worrying about sicknesses that are related to seasonal changes.

Since we've already talked about the dietary habits, now is a good time to discuss various yoga practices that benefit you in different seasons. There's a huge misconception that yoga is all about asanas, and nothing else. However, that's not true. Yoga is much more than that. There are a lot of practices involved here, which help you stay healthy, both physically and mentally. Let's start with the winter yoga practices.

Winter Yoga Practices

Even though winter seems like a pretty good season, you may not feel the same throughout the season, since, come one, who likes to spend their days, shivering out, burning too many calories, while staying at home all day?! Add to that, there are several common and prevalent sicknesses related to this season. So, here are a few tips for you to follow:

Stay warm: You may be tempted to sleep longer than usual, as it feels nice and cozy, almost every winter morning.

However, you're doing only harm to yourself. As sleeping longer, usually leads you avoid the Yoga session, you're missing out on one of the best practices that help you keep warm. Yes, yoga can immensely help you in staying warm.

Beat the bacteria: How can you beat something that you can't see? Alright, I admit, it was a bad joke. But hey, you can really defeat bacteria and the related infections with yoga and an Ayurvedic diet. Regular yoga helps you strengthen your immune system. But, it goes beyond that. If you're interested in doing advanced yoga, you'll be hugely benefited. For example, pranayamas, the yogic breathing exercises, makes it easy for you to handle chest congestion. It also helps you fight off the common winter allergies and infections, which are caused by bacteria.

Meditate for a better mind: I can't stress enough on how important it is to meditate in Winters, especially if you're suffering from anxiety and depression. See, Winter is a season where the weather is all gloomy and dark. And, what does it do to our mind?! Dark and gloomy climate can turn your mood into the same, making it all more difficult to deal with mental health issues. Here, a good session of calm and focused meditation could go a long way. So, please try to follow this tip with utmost importance.

Eat, but eat healthily: In winters, it's quite natural that your body turns on the shivering mechanism to cope with the cold climate around you. While doing so, your body also burns out a lot of calories, very fast. So, it's important that you supply the body with enough food, so that it doesn't go out of the fuel supplies to function properly. But hey, don't take advantage of the situation and go on a binge session of junk food. Always make sure that you stress on healthy food intake.

Summer Yoga Practices

Summer, with its warm, sometimes too hot weather, is a great time to spend, with your family. First, you don't have to worry about not being able to go out, since you don't have to deal with issues such as rain or snow. And then, Summer also wards off a lot of bacterial infections, since the sun kills them all with brutal UV rays. However, it also affects us, which is why we need to follow a few practices, that are specifically custom-tailored for this season. Here are a few Ayurvedic practices for you to follow in Summertime.

Focus on your breath: Oh! I'm not talking about your usual breath. However, I'm talking about the infamous Ayurvedic breathing exercises, pranayamas. In Summer, particularly, sheetali pranayama works wonders. It's quite easy to do, and is very effective. Start by sticking out your tongue, as if you're trying to whistle. Then, slowly breathe in, through your mouth, and hold it for a few seconds, and then breathe out through your nose. Do this for 5 to 10 times a day, as it helps you cool down your body's temperature.

Drink it up: I'm very sure that you may have already known how important it is to stay hydrated in Summer. Well, you could do a bit better than that. As the scorching heat in the summers are sometimes unforgiving, you need to do a little more than just drinking water. Along with taking gallons of water, try following the sheetkari pranayama. Clench your teeth, while your mouth open, and then press your tongue against your teeth. Now, take a deep breath. Hold it for a few seconds, and then breathe it out through your nose. This practice helps you deal with unending thirst, which is a usual thing in Summer.

Stay calm and stay cool: The summer heat makes you tired and restless, which, in turn affects your mood as well. This is especially true for the people who're dealing with mental health issues. So, here's a simple solution for you to stay calm and composed. chandrabhedi could help you by leaps and bounds here. With your right thumb, close your right nostril. Use your left nostril to exhale and then to inhale. Close your left nostril using the left little finger. Repeat the inhalation and exhalation process, but with your right nostril. Do this 5-10 times a day.

Monsoon Yoga Practices

Since we're done with Summer and Winter, we now move to less intense seasons such as Monsoon. Who don't love going for a morning walk in a Monsoon? I mean, I'd say Monsoon is the best season, with perfect balance of the temperatures, climate, and overall conditions which are not too good or too bad. However, with Monsoons, there's an overwhelmingly common risk of cold and flu. Now, you know what to do, right? Learn some yoga practices that are perfectly designed for such season, and implement them. Here are a few tips for you to stay balanced and healthy in this season.

Take care of the respiratory tract: The common flu and cold infections target your respiratory system. Without proper care, the situation could sometimes go out of control. But, don't you worry about that. Simply follow the kapal bhati pranayama, and all your respiratory tract problems go away, just like that. It's also called the "Breath of Fire." Sit comfortably, erect your spine, and place your hands on the knees. Inhale while pulling your navel back to the spine. Hold it for a couple of seconds, and then exhale while relaxing your belly. Do it a few times every day.

Take care of your sinuses: Sinusitis is such a huge issue, especially if you're suffering from anxiety or depression. It not only makes it difficult to breath properly, but also negatively impacts your mood and mindset. To avoid such issues, simply go for the nadi shodhan pranayama. It helps you open up your blocked nostrils, and at the same time improves your sinus resistance. Sit in a comfortable manner with your spine erect. Relax your shoulders, and keep your left hand on the knee. Keep your right index finger and middle finger between your eyebrows. Use your ring finger and little finger to open and close your nostrils. Now, breathe in, with a nostril closed, and breathe out through the other nostril. Repeat it with both the nostrils few times a day. Voila!

Fall Yoga Practices

The most beautiful of the seasons, and also the most endearing of all, the Fall. Usually, you might find yourself, chilling and enjoying the weather in this season. But, you should take it up to the next level. Oh, I'm taking about taking advantage of this amazing season to heal your mental health issues. As the beauty of this season already calms your mind, you should try implementing a few yoga practices to get the full benefit out of it. So, without any further ado, here are a few yoga practices for the Fall.

Cleanse your body and mind: In the beauty of mother nature in its fully glory, why not take some time and focus on cleaning your whole body and mind?! Yep, it's still legal to do that. Kapalbhati, which means "shining skull," is an amazingly effective method to take care of your entire body system. By doing this, you can remove all the toxins from your body and mind. Sit cross-legged and set your spine straight. Now, inhale a deep breath and hold it for a couple of seconds. Then, force it out in a short and rapid burst of exhalation. Repeat it for 20 times continuously to get the most out of it.

Stay balanced and composed: Well, easier said than done, isn't it? Yes, I can understand your frustration. While dealing with any mental health issue, staying composed is one of the most difficult things. But, there's always a way! Vrikshasana, which also known as the "tree pose," is the thing you need in your life, if you're looking to stay balanced. It's a yoga posture which requires balance and focus. Stand still and bend the right knee, and then keep your right foot on the left thigh. Keep your left leg straight. Put your palms in the 'Namaste' pose. Now, it's time to take a strong and deep breath. Hold the breath for 5-10 seconds before releasing it through slow exhalation.

Food and the Mind: Understanding the Mind-Body Connection

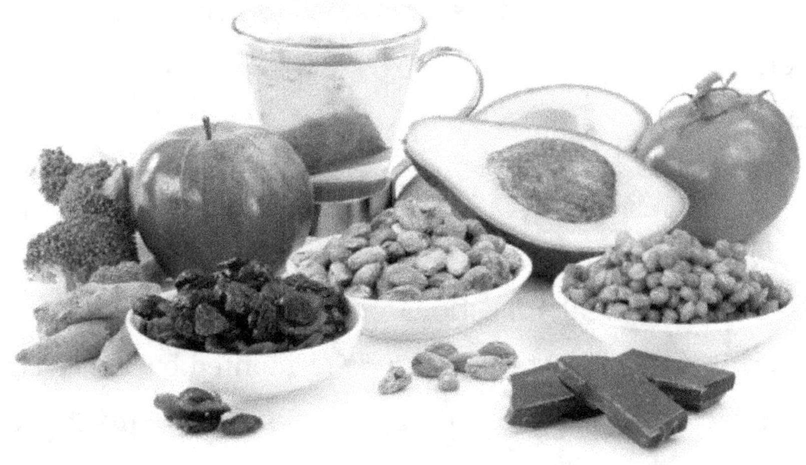

According to Ayurveda, there are three major junctions, aka maha marmas. They come between consciousness and physiology. One is located in the head called shiras marma, and the other is located in the heart called hridaya marma, and the last one in the bladder is called basti marma. All three of them have their own (agni) fire, metabolism and functions. The agni of the head is called medo agni that regulates intelligence. Agni of heart is smriti agni, that regulates memory. Agni of the lower pelvic area is called prajanana agni. When food goes through this agni, functions like digestion and transformation in balance, it nourishes the whole physiology creating balance in the mind, heart, and regenerative functions of the body. Body and mind are interconnected in a such a way that when these three marmas are in their balanced state, we tend to think clearer, experience happiness, have refined awareness, and balanced emotions.

Better Digestion, Better Mood

When we have weak digestion, food stays in stomach for longer times and start to rot due to fermented bacteria. This rotten food along with bacteria produces endotoxins that are poisonous to our whole body system. This poison in Ayurveda is ama.

Negative experiences including grief, loss, trauma, or any other PTSD symptoms may trigger anxiety or depression. Such things could also stay intact in your mind, which also has high chances of creating troubles in the future.

Ama and Mood

Over a period of time, this mental ama gets accumulated and can influence our quality of life. we feel worthless, uninspired, exhausted and drab. It leads to stagnation of bodily channels and our emotions trapped in mind leading to suppression. The relation of brain and our tummy is a two-way street; messages from gut travel upriver with the help of the vagus nerve. The gut has more information that needs to reach the brain. The microbes in our GI tract produce neurotransmitters and have control on our brain.

Specific cells in our gut have control on our mood by producing hormones like serotonin- the happy hormone and neurochemical endorphin - that gives us euphoria feeling. When there is ama, it irritates our gut and toxins are released into blood stream, and irritate our nervous system and play with our emotions.

Ayurvedic Tricks for a Better Mind

These simple Ayurvedic tricks are a way to bump off anxiety, relieve stress, and change your current mood from feeling drab to happy.

Write

Write something you would love to do now instead of what you are currently doing.

Feeling low and lethargic sometimes? Would you like a sudden transition from things you are currently doing to things you would rather love to do? I say pen it down, be it going for a movie or being with your loved ones, or any activity that you would love to do. Write them down.

Sip on Herbal Tea

Herbal teas can help us avoid feeling edgy with stress and anxiety and can also be used as a routine complementary therapy. Carry these herbal tea bags and indulge in them when anxiety kicks in. It's important to realize that herbal teas that work for one person may not work for all. So, finding the right blend of herbs can take time. But I'll tell you herbs and the situations where they helped people according to research. The aroma of peppermint oil may reduce anxiety, frustration and fatigue. Some research showed that it helped soothe anxiety in hospitalized people for pregnancy (childbirth) and heart attack. Chamomile helps people with a generalized anxiety disorder. Lavender is famous for its mood-stabilizing ability, along with sedative effects. Another research showed that oral lavender capsule preparation (silexan) was equally effective as lorazepam for people suffering from generalized anxiety disorder. Lemon balm is known to help in insomnia, anxiety, depression in patients suffering from heart condition called Angina. It boosts a neuro transmitter that soothes stress called GABA receptors. Green tea has high amount of amino acid, l-theanine that reduces anxiety.

Shake Off While You Stand

Stand up and keep feet firmly on to the ground. Now lift one leg at a time and shake your leg while you breathe in and out thrice. Try to balance but if it's difficult then hold on to a chair. After shaking both legs, shake your hands for good three breaths. Shaking releases our stiff muscles and awakens our inner connection, like we restart our slow computer, this technique helps in restarting our nervous system that's been undergoing involuntary shaking, this sends mood-enhancing signals from shaking muscles directly to the central nervous system.

The 6 Tastes of Food

Here, I'll explain pretty much everything about the six tastes of food, their significance, qualities, benefits, and everything else there is to discuss. According to Ayurveda, the person who eats all these 6 tastes in balance succeeds in maintaining a very healthy life. Although Ayurveda is a 5000-year-old science, its approach towards taste is unique and scientific, since each of the tastes have their own therapeutic effects and impact on our body. Our taste buds do so much more than just identifying tastes, they unlock the goodness of nutrition and kick start to break down foods. Foods that we consume travel from tip of our tongue till getting absorbed by the body, ayurvedic diet distinguishes them into six tastes/rasas.

The six tastes are sweet, sour, salty, bitter, pungent, and astringent.

Sweet taste is our taste buds favorite and comes through naturally-occurring sugars. it's a flavor of energy and they nourish us. Foods and herbs that have sweet flavor in them fall in this category. Food sources are carbohydrates, proteins and fats like rice, grains, licorice, pasta, bread, meat, fish, dairy, chicken and starchy vegetables, sweet fruits, beet root, carrot, honey, and sugar.

Salt is the taste that enhances any taste of food and is a flavor that creates moisture and heat in our body. Mineral salts, seaweed, fish, soy sauce, tasting salt, salted meats come under this category.

In India, sour and unripe fruits are made into pickles and consumed with curd rice in every meal as digestive pickles. We tend to salivate with the sight of sour foods and they also stimulate digestion. Fruits that are sour in taste are citrus fruits, fermented foods, sauerkraut, sourdough, breads, milk products like sour cream, cheese, and yoghurt. Pickles, vinegar, and wine are some sour foods.

With pungent (spicy) food, our tongue doesn't have any specific receptors to perceive spicy taste. It is perceived through tissue irritation and nerve endings. Peppers, cloves, chilies, garlic, onions, wasabi, spices, mustard, black pepper, ginger, salsa, cayenne, radish, cardamom are some good examples. They clear congestion, remove mucus, and are warming. They also boost metabolism.

If you ever wondered why green leafy veggies taste Bitter, it's like defense mechanism, if they taste bitter, no one would eat them. They contain alkaloids and glycosides, veggies like Spinach, celery, kale, aubergine (eggplant), sprouts, broccoli, beets, courgetti (zucchini), spices like dandelion, turmeric, and fenugreek. Fruits like bitter melons, grapefruits, and olives.

Have you ever tried eating unripe bananas or cranberries, or that overstepping tea bags leave your tea and taste buds with sharp bitter flavors? The reason behind that is tannins, and that weird taste is astringent. It makes your mouth contract and pulls the mucus membranes together. It is found in plants as compounds called tannins food sources such as lentils, beans and fruits like cranberries, pears, green apples, pomegranates. vegetables like broccoli, cauliflower, cabbage artichoke, dried beans, asparagus and turnip. grains like rye, quinoa, buckwheat. spices like turmeric and marjoram. Tannins are in high amount in coffee, tea, dry crackers, and some raw vegetables and fruit skins like grape skin. Astringent taste helps n wound healing and during fluid retention and swelling in the body.

According to Ayurveda, these 6 tastes in our dietary habits meet the needs, and are building blocks of body. For example, sweet foods are rich in proteins, carbohydrates, water, and fats. Whereas foods that are Bitter and Astringent are abundant in vitamins and minerals. Foods that are salty encourages stability and good for nervous system. Our brain has messenger pathways that sends signals to our body when in need of energy through food. When you incorporate these 6 tastes in every meal, we can be rest assured that these signals are met adequately. This in turn suppresses food cravings and overeating habit. This tabular column below shows the physical and mental effects when consumed adequately and excessively for all six tastes.

Crafting a Balanced Menu

There's this famous saying, "We are what we eat", and that goes just beyond physical health and body. Now, what's health if it's only about being physically well? It's how you feel in your head too. As mentioned earlier, the food we eat is intimately connected with how we feel and think in mind. That is, mental and emotional health. Of course, in order to lead healthy life, you just don't need balance in structural and bodily functions like digestion, metabolism and excretion, but also attain self-awareness with senses and mind.

Using the principles of ayurvedic nutrition, a balanced meal means having six tastes in each meal that nourishes and satisfies the body. Make food choices from the following food examples.

Compatible and Incompatible Food Combinations

1. Fruits are best eaten alone and at least 30 minutes before any meal or at least 2 hours post meal. Remember, this is possibly the most important food rule among all.

2. Eggs are incompatible with fruits, most importantly melons, and beans, cheese, kitchari (a dish made of rice and legumes), fish, meat, milk, and yoghurt.

3. Legumes are incompatible with fruits, milk, cheese, fish, eggs, yoghurt. Legumes are best eaten with starches like rice to make it a perfect protein combo.

4. Grains are incompatible with fruits and tapioca.

5. Concerning honey, the first rule of thumb is honey should never be heated or undergo any form of cooking like baking or boiling, because the molecules in honey become unrecognizable to the body making it indigestible. Mixing honey with ghee is also toxic.

6. Lemon is incompatible with cucumber, yoghurt, tomatoes, and milk.

7. Nightshades like eggplants, potatoes, tomatoes, peppers, tomatillos, and tobacco are incompatible with cucumber, melon, and dairy products. In inflammatory conditions like arthritis and irritable bowel syndrome, this rule must be followed with high priority.

8. Starches and grains are incompatible with proteins and sugary foods.

9. Vegetables are incompatible with fruits and raw veggies doesn't go well with cooked veggies. But they go well with starches and proteins.

10. Yoghurt is incompatible with fruits, eggs, fish, cheese, milk, meat, and nightshades.

11. Proteins are incompatible with other source of proteins, eat protein of one source at a time as different proteins require different enzymes to digest, also avoid high fat foods as they inhibit the synthesis of necessary enzymes that are needed for digestion of proteins. Proteins are also incompatible with starchy foods and high carbohydrate

foods.

12. Tapioca is incompatible with fruits, importantly bananas, mangoes and beans, japery, and raisins

13. Use spices and condiments to boost your immunity and healing properties that food has to offer.

14. Consideration of diurnal and seasonal changes

There's a three-way conversation between our gut, brain and microbiota of gastrointestinal tract. A wide range of choices that we make have an impact on our microbiota like foods we eat, medicines and supplements, amount of sleep we get, diseases, stress, and environment you live in, and what time we eat and our eating window, that is the time interval between your meals. Our health is dependent on microbiota largely. The state of our microbiota has impact on our immune system, digestive system, metabolic system, neurological system, and overall wellbeing. Researchers have proved that the microbiota is more active during daytime than at night, making it diurnal.

Our body and brain are diurnal too. Our human brain has internal light meters and clock proteins in almost every cell.

Sleep and wake cycles are controlled by light hours and dark hours of the day. It communicates with the central nervous system and body's master gland-pituitary gland; it is called so because it controls other hormones of body. Here CNS and pituitary gland put effects on endocrine glands (hormones) and other systems. So they have control of our mood.

Eat According to Time and Season

In ancient times, humans ate only once or twice, as the maximum used to be two meals a day. Its mentioned in ayurvedic texts that two meals a day was the ideal number one should de consuming.

According to Ayurveda, the limit of two meals a day and the water we drink is connected to excretory functions. It is advised that one can have 2-3 bowel movements in a day and urinating 6 times a day.

As per Ayurveda, a day has two pitta dominant dayparts, 10 am- 2pm in the morning, and during the night, it is from 10 pm - 2 am. The morning pitta peaks around at 12 noon precisely, and the night pitta at 12 in the midnight. Due to the absence of the sun at night, the night pitta at 12 pm is considered to be dampening. And the ability of our digestive system is much weaker post-sunset. So making the digestive fire at 12 noon the most ideal and stronger one.

So, we should consider eating our large meal for lunch and the lightest meal for dinner. By this we help our body digest easily and it will thank us in return, by absorbing all nutrients and retaining them. As we all know, it takes our body 3-4 hours to digest each full meal. It might take longer if the food is heavy and our digestive fire is weak. You can eat fruits, snacks in between meals only if you are hungry.

Don't just simply eat because someone told you to eat 6 meals a day as a health tip. We are not cows to graze, they chew their cuds all the time, as all grazing animals have totally different digestive systems, and that's a whole different story. So let's not get inspired by them.

Now coming to the seasonal changes, in seasons with lengthy nights and short days, one must consume food only in the morning. In seasons with lengthy days and short nights, one must consume the food during sunset and during afternoons.

If you ever wondered how much to eat, you should consider your age, body type and doshas, current season, doshic balance and imbalance, type of exercise, and the type of food you are consuming. Rule of thumb of Ayurveda is to eat food half of our capacity, drink water one-fourth of our capacity, and leave space of one-fourth capacity for food to move freely and digest easily.

One should feel satisfied, but not heavy, after a meal. One should be able to breathe normally, walk, and talk easily after meal.

Eat foods once you have excreted stool and urine. Walk when you feel your body light and mind pleasant and clear. The stomach should be empty, clear and light. When hunger strikes, you will develop an interest to consume food. Now the body will receive food happily and digest properly and utilize nutrients to our body.

Addressing Digestive Imbalances

In India, from ancient ayurvedic times, wheat was consumed as a staple comfort cereal. Even today, wheat is consumed on a daily basis and Ayurveda recommends using wheat on a daily basis. Gluten is a protein from grains like wheat, rye, barley and spelt. Among all these gluten containing grains, the most commonly consumed one is wheat.

According to Ayurveda, gluten intolerance is a type of ajeerna/indigestion. Symptoms manifest based on a person's dominant dosha. Coeliac disease is severe form of gluten intolerance. Statistics from 2013 stated that more than three million people in America suffer from celiac disease, that is approximately 1 in 133 people. However, recent stats suggest the number is closer to one in hundred. As per the 2013 survey, a third of Americans consciously avoid gluten.

In patients with celiac disease, the immune system thinks that the gluten proteins are foreign invaders, and activates defense mechanism and causes inflammation that in turn damages intestinal lining and malabsorption of nutrients. Symptoms in vata dominant person along with gluten intolerance can have bloating, headache, abdominal colic pain, lastly weight loss and tiredness over a period of time. Whereas pitta dominant types can manifest symptoms like pain in abdominal colic, diarrhea with smelly feces. Lastly if kaphna dominant types is gluten intolerant they can have symptoms like feeling heavy, skin allergies, and depression.

Ayurvedic way of treatment includes using spices like asfoetida, fenugreek, black cumin, black pepper, cumin, turmeric, long pepper. Herbal teas to help wheat intolerance are triphala, amalaki, guduchi, bilva, and psyllium seed fiber supplement. Followed by panchakarma detoxification therapy based on your doshic imbalances.

Lactose intolerance is when your body lacks the ability to process and digest lactose, which is a form of sugar. Lactose is usually found in milk and some other dairy products. People with lactose intolerance feel uncomfortableness in their stomach, along with bloating and pain. There are several herbs you can take to deal with this condition. Here are a few things that could help you.

Bilva: This herb stimulates your digestive fire, in turn helping you combat diarrhea, which is a common symptom of lactose intolerance.

Vaividang: It helps you reduce the nausea, which is also another common symptom of the lactose intolerance.

Daruharidra: A herb that can help you improve the overall metabolic and digestive systems of your body.

Kutaj: An infamous herb that's used to treat lactose intolerance. It produces an antispasmodic action, which in turn helps you reduce cramps and pain in the abdomen.

Ayurvedic Diet Seasonal Guides

Ayurveda considers having a seasonal routine year around is important and as a backbone of our health. Balancing the changes in nature of our climate with form of living that counterbalance the form of imbalances that are seasonally-induced is one of the simplest ways to protect our well-being. An interesting fact is that our body and mind adapt to habits that are appropriate for particular seasons without even us being conscious of picking those. For example, we often tend to enjoy fresh salads and consume lots of watermelons in summer; they both work as perfect antidotes to beat that choking summer heat. Whereas from October and November, baking season is officially set to begin with pies, pumpkin bread and baked potatoes, grounding soups. Dining on hearty foods that naturally suppress the light, dry nature of the fall. By making changes in dietary habits and lifestyle choices to counterbalance the effects of four seasons, we can have better health and maintain the internal sense of equilibrium around the year.

Autumn is the classic vata season. According to Ayurveda by simply increasing the opposites we can stay balanced. for example, we feel extremely cold, dry, light, windy and totally unpredictable during fall season. To make it less aggravating we need to fill in warmth, oiliness, nourish deeply, loving relationships, and a routine sense of stability and groundedness.

Autumn/Vata Season Diet

Our diet is the only major way to soothe vata this fall season. Substantive and oily, nourishing foods that have high amounts of protein and fats in them, cooking them with warming and heat stimulating spices, and serving them hot, goes a long way in maintaining our body with moisture and helps you stay grounded throughout the vata season. You might want to favor tastes like sweet, sour, and salty. Eat soft mushy foods and add your favorite herbs like thyme, basil, rosemary or use lemon for fish and seafood or to make it ayurvedic way use ghee or mustard oil and garnish them generously. Breakfasts made of cooked grains suck as tapioca, oatmeal, cream of rice, and wheat make perfect choice for this time of year. include steamed veggies, soups, stews and broths, hearty grains that are extremely grounding and add warmth and moisture to our body as a meal for a lunch or dinner.

If you love eggs and meat than this season is for you, fall is best time to savor them, indulge in healthful dairy and crunchy nuts and seeds to benefit during fall. In general, you should reduce your consumption of chilled beverages, ice creams, frozen foods, raw veggies, along with the pungent, bitter and astringent tastes. It is better to minimize intake of light, drying and cooling foods like cabbage, cauliflower, broccoli, sprouts, white potatoes, beans, leafy greens, popcorn, millets, crackers and dried fruits. If you are someone who can resist these foods that are supposed to be avoided for this season its totally okay to consume them in moderation, but make sure to cook them well and soak them well, and serve them with ghee for added extra benefits.

During the fall season you may end up eating a lot; it's natural for us to increase the intake of food but try to listen to your body and takes its lead for appetite and digestion. You might feel hungry very often during fall and it requires proper nourishment so its best time to do monotype diet for cleansing. I hope you found it helpful to become familiar with your body and the signs and symptoms of imbalance in vata, so that you are well prepared to tackle any issues immediately, just in case if they arise. These recommendations go with most of the people, but if you are aware of your constitution and state of balance you need to achieve currently, you can modify or customize your seasonal routines accordingly.

Fruits: bananas, grapes, cooked apples, avocados, dates, lemons, oranges, soaked prunes, tangerines, soaked tangerines, soaked raisins, figs, limes, papayas, mangoes

Vegetables: garlic, ladies finger, beets, carrots, onions, chilies, winter squash, sweet potatoes, and pumpkins

Dairy: ghee, butter, cream, sour cream, buttermilk, warm milk, kefir, yoghurt, cheese

Legumes: kidney beans, split black gram, miso, green gram, pigeon peas

Nuts and seeds: you can consume all kinds of nuts during this season

Animal products: eggs, beef, duck, buffalo, chicken, turkey, venison, seafood like shrimp, oysters, fish, lobster

Grains: basmati rice, oats, amaranth, wheat, brown rice, quinoa

Oils: almond oil, olive oil, peanut oil, sesame oil, ghee

Sweeteners: raw sugar, rice syrup, maple syrup, molasses, honey, jaggery

Spices: All spices are good to consume during this season, including turmeric, black pepper, anise, cardamom, nutmeg, cinnamon, asafoetida, cumin, rosemary, ginger, bay leaf, basil, mustard seeds, ginger, parsley, oregano, saffron, paprika

Herbal support for fall: To boost immunity, consume chyavanprash everyday in the morning. it can help boost immunity improve strength, and energy. Ashwagandha helps in stabilizing the mind and nervous system, and can help in promoting sound sleep, proper digestion, elimination, chyavanprash is available in the form of a powder, liquid extract and tablet. Herbal teas made of ginger, cumin, fennel and coriander combined with licorice can help in proper digestion and add warmth to our body. Some vitalizing herbs and their formulas are dashamula, haritaki, triphala, which are also available in the form of tablets and vidari. These herbs are quite supporting during fall.

Summer/Pitta Season Diet

This spectacular season with bright sun and long days and its transformative nature go hand in hand with pitta, which is why summer is thought to be the pitta season.

Summer is when our bodies by default want light foods and tiny meals that are highly digestible to keep us cool because the digestive fire being the strong source of internal heat, it diffuses for the same purpose, to keep us cool. As I mentioned earlier mindful eating can help one with overeating, being in presence with your food while savoring, you will enjoy its flavor and texture of your food that will in return stop us from overeating. Summer is a good time to eat flavors that are sweet, astringent and bitter. It's the best time to savor cool, fresh fruits, juices and salads. Indulge in dairy products such as milk, ghee, cottage cheese, butter, homemade yogurt and ice cream. Avoid honey and molasses and savor all kinds of unrefined sweeteners in moderation as they are cooling to our body.

When it comes to drinking cold drinks to beat the heat, try to consume infused water that has mint, lime and raw sugar or herbal teas like licorice, peppermint, fennel or rose and sweet lassi. Do not add ice cubes, it's best to avoid iced drinks as they disturb our digestive fire and let toxins buildup in our body. Go easy on oily foods, sour fruits or unripe fruits, spices, aged cheeses, and do not cook vegetables like carrots, beets, onions, radishes, garlic, mustard seeds, and ginger. Avoid chilies, cayenne pepper, and hot chili sauces. Also, keep in mind that salads with raw veggies are better digested when eaten for lunch instead of dinner.

Fruits: apples, grapes, avocados, limes, plums, pomegranates, coconuts, cherries, cranberries, mangoes, berries, melons, prunes, pears, and pineapples

Vegetables: asparagus, collard greens, artichokes, beet greens, cabbage, cauliflower, brussels sprouts, kale, chard, lettuce, okra, chard, watercress, green beans, cucumber, celery

Grains: basmati, wheat, rice, barley

Legumes: soybeans and its products, red mung beans, chickpeas, mung beans, split peas, black beans

Oils: coconut oil, sunflower oil, olive oil

Spices and garnishes: cardamom, fennel, coriander, dill, basil, cilantro, mint, lime, parsley

Animal products: freshwater fish, shrimp, white poultry meat

Sweeteners: turbinado, maple syrup, jaggery

Spring Season Diet

Spring is the season of less cold, warmth, moisture. During spring, there is an increased heaviness of moisture. Our cravings naturally shift as winter passes, and spring arrives. Our appetite decreases, and we crave for fruits, fresh vegetables and salads. Since warmer weather has arrived our desire to eat heavy foods that were essential earlier for winter decreases. This is our body's way of telling us that it's time for detoxifying and cleansing our body. This season is a perfect time for juice fasts. People in ancient India used fresh acidic juices to help with fatigue and prevent many ailments. Limes were believed to be sacred according to the Vedas because of its ability to cleanse and purify the human body. This season is extremely supportive for Juice fasts with apple juice, pomegranate or liquid diets with soups, smoothies and juices, or monodiets.

Along with dietary cleanse, our body has a natural desire to rejuvenate, you can help your body with this by favoring the bitter, pungent, astringent flavors and by eating light, warm foods that are highly digestible. These dietary habits control moisture levels, balance mucus production in body and open the channels for toxin elimination and aiding in purification. Moreover, you can promote health by warm, hot beverages or at least at room temperatures. Consider drinking some warm water with a dollop of honey during the day. Eat lots of fresh steamed veggies and legumes since they have astringent and bitter flavors. You can never go wrong with veggies, but make sure not to overdo veggies that have abundance of water in them like cucumber, squash, zucchini or buttery avocados, sweet potatoes and olives.

Start your day with fruits for breakfast and tea, that's light on our tummy. Steamed veggies, cooked grains, legumes make perfect choice for lunches and dinners. Eat veggies like broccoli, cabbage, cauliflower and bitter greens and spicy green chilies and lots of bitter greens. Eat in moderate or avoid hardboiled or poached eggs, tofu and freshwater fish during spring season. Add foods with pungent flavors like garlic, black pepper, onions, ginger, bell peppers, cayenne peppers in small amounts and lots of spices and herbs. Alongside reduce consuming oily, fried or heavy foods gradually. Practice mindful eating and don't overeat, or snack in between meals. Try to consume sweet, salty and sour flavors in moderation.

Fruits that are heavy like bananas, coconuts, dates, figs and sour fruits like oranges, melons and pineapples are best reduced. Reduce intake of dairy, especially during mornings as they can cause congestion. Substitute dairy with almond milk or rice milk. If you are habituated to drinking cow's milk, boil it and cool it down and drink it warm by adding grated ginger or pinch of turmeric to make it easily digestible. Eating adequately and more frequently the meat like pork, beef, duck, seafood can help us during this season. Avoid junk, fast foods, nuts, sweets, soy products, bread, and frozen or chilled foods. If possible try to eliminate ice cream, chilled beverages, and popsicles.

Fruits: apples, cherries, apricots, cranberries, blueberries, pears, dried fruits, peaches, lemons, pomegranates, limes, strawberries, soaked prunes, raspberries and raisins

Vegetables: lettuce, artichoke, mushrooms, asparagus, chard, chilies, bell pepers, onions, collard greens, dandelion greens, beets and beet, corn, broccoli, peas, endive, radishes, kale, potatoes, garlic, sprouts, brussels sprouts, spinach, carrots, kale, cabbage, turnips, green beans, leeks, celery, cauliflower

Grains: barley, quinoa, amaranth, corn, tapioca, rice cakes, dry oats (don't cook), millets, buckwheat, seitan, rye, basmati rice

Winter/Kapha Diet

Winter has a sense of heaviness due to cold weather, increased moisture usually by rain or snow, cloudy days, season of hibernation for many animals. Gives us slow feels and groundedness.

Our digestive fire is strongest during winters. our body needs more fuel during winters to warm up and keep our body healthy, due to increased digestive fire there is increased appetite and you will likely end up eating larger portion of food. Our bodies crave for substantial, nutritious diet during this time. Winter diet should be aimed at pacifying kapha. Winter dietary habits comes quite naturally as we tend to focus on consuming warm, cooked food that is well spiced and slightly oily and favoring all six tastes in each meal.

Drink beverages at warm, hot or at room temperature, avoid chilled drinks, ice creams. By drinking herbal teas we can increase heat circulation in body and clears respiratory blockages. ever heard of the Ayurveda's miracle tea called

CCF Tea. Add Water and half spoon of each dried ginger, cinnamon and clove boil for five minutes. Sip on this CCF tea throughout the day or after meals. This tea is a game changer when it comes to improving digestion. Vegetables that increases body temperature like radish, carrots, onions, spinach, root veggies are a good choice during this season. Hot spices like ginger, chili peppers, cayenne, garlic and black peppers are well received by our body and boost immunity during this flu season.

Cooking your grains like barley, tapioca, rice, cornmeal, oatmeal or making kitchari is a fabulous choice for breakfast. Steamed veggies, mushy soups and whole wheat breads are ideal during this season. Legumes that are well cooked and well spiced, garnished with some ghee are good for kapha as they don't aggravate vata. Winter is a great time to eat animal protein like eggs that are poached or hardboiled and chicken, venison, turkey, and rabbit.

It's best to avoid dairy during winters but a cup of spiced hot milk with a little turmeric or nutmeg or dried ginger before bed can put us to sleep and improve quality of sleep over time. But should not be overdone, as it may cause congestion.

Ayurvedic Kitchen Basics

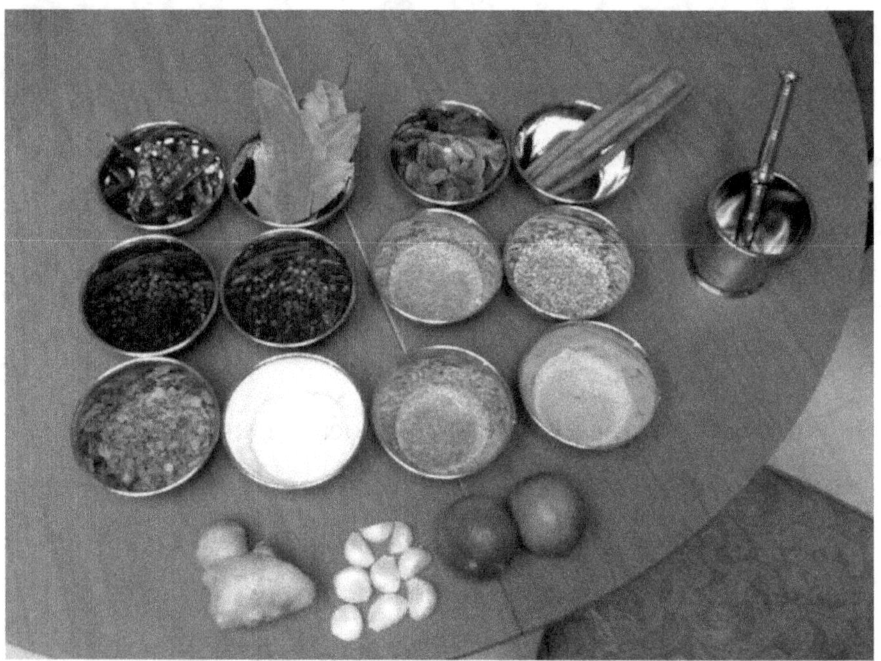

Chyawanprash

Chyawanprash is an ancient ayurvedic health supplement. that is a super concentrated blend inclusive of a rich nutritive herbs and minerals. It is known to revive ojas (drained life forces) and to conserve strength, energy and vitality, while delaying the aging process.

The ayurvedic recipe of chyawanprash is cited in

manuscripts written in ashtanga hridya, charaka samita and sangandhara samita. Amla/Indian gooseberry being the key ingredient in making of chyawanprash, it is rich in vitamin C with (445 mg/100g). Chyawanprash has been a staple in India for 5000 years and Indians consider it their tradition as an effective food supplement and three course meal with zeal and vitality, and has lived owing to its incredible health care benefits. According to ancient ayurvedic texts around 25 -80 kind of herbs go into this miracle recipe. It is cooked with mixture of honey, ghee, (amla jam) Indian gooseberry, sugar, berries, sesame oil, many herbs and spices make this powerful recipe.

Preparation of chyawanprash is done according to instruction suggested in ayurvedic texts. Chyawanprash is readily available in India and days these brands make them in many fruity flavors and sugar free for diabetics. It is sold in large scale and consumed largely in India as a regular nutritional supplement.

Chyawanprash is a preparation formulated by processing amla (Indian gooseberry) as a prime ingredient; alma is richest source of vitamin C among all, nearly 50 medicinal herbs and their extracts go into its making. These herbs are used by preparing a dried extract and decoction and further mixed with honey, and adding aromatic herbal powders made of spices like clove, cinnamon, and cardamom. The final product is in consistency of fruit jam and has flavors of sweet, sour, and spicy. Base paste of chyawanprash consists of amla/Indian gooseberry pulp. This is known as the most efficient rasayana that supports homeostasis.

Nutritional Facts and Usage

Chyawanprash can be used by everyone in every season, the ingredients eliminate the unpleasant effects of environmental changes around us. The normal dosage of (12–28 g) can be taken with 100- 250 ml of milk on an empty stomach in the morning.

Chyawanprash is reported to be rich in vitamins, proteins, dietary fibers, carbohydrates, and low fat contents (no-trans and zero percent cholesterol), major and minor trace metals in (mg/100g), such as iron (21.1), zinc (3.1), cobalt (3.7), copper (0.667), nickel (1.4), magnesium (8.3), vitamin C (0.5), tannic acid (20.2), other vitamins such as A, B1, B2, E and micronutrients like carotenoids, flavonoids, alkaloids, antioxidants, saponins, phenolic compounds, piperine, etc. Rich formula of vitamin C, E along with carotenoids, antioxidants, and its powerful nutritional composition is known for synergistic effects work as immuno-modulator, body building and in restoring health along with preventing the oxidative damage that leads to degenerative diseases.

Chyawanprash enhances the calcium absorption and protein synthesis, making our bones and teeth strong, and our muscles toned. This rasayana has intense effect in growth and to gain weight due to effective herbs like guduchi, ashwagandha, and fruit amla helping in balancing the body's natural process and regulate the neuroendocrine-immune activity. It detoxifies blood and eliminates impurities. It promotes pilosity of hair and improves skin complexion, cures dermal infections, and leaves you with youthfulness, vitality, and glowing skin.

A study conducted to evaluate benefits of chyawanprash for health promotion in elderly people showed a decrease in cholesterol levels, LDL (low-density lipoprotein), triglycerides and increased the HDL (high-density lipoprotein) levels which confirms its support in improving health in elderly its beneficial effects and indications of this formulation in geriatrics.

Content of Chyawanprash

ashwagandha (Winter cherry)

asparagus racemose

amla

bamboo manna

cinnamon bark

makhana (fox nuts) of blue Egyptian water lily

cardamom

chebulic myrobalan

clove

Chinese cinnamon

Indian rose chestnut

galls

country mallow

feather foil plant (Phyllanthus niruri)

ghee

giant potato (Ipomoea mauritiana)

(Guduchi) (Tinospora cordifolia)

honey

Indian kudzu

long pepper (Piper longum)

Irish root

Malabar nut (Seed of Adhatoda vasica)

nut grass

raisins

potassium sorbate

round zedoary

sesame oil

sandalwood

punarnava (Spreading hogweed)

sugar

Indian coral tree (Erythrina variegata)

wild black and green gram

Ayurvedic Must-Have Herbs in Your Kitchen

Curry Leaves

This one is a staple in every Indian kitchen for its

tremendous health benefits. They are known for anti-diabetic, anti-inflammatory, antioxidant, antimicrobial, anti-carcinogenic, mild laxative properties, and also protects liver (hepatoprotective properties) in it. Add them to your salad to reap its benefits.

Brahmi

This herb was called as elixir in ancient ayurvedic texts for its enormous benefits. It's known for its anti-inflammatory, anticancer, and antioxidant properties. It stands out among all the herbs when treating anxiety, because it targets the stress hormone and reduces its secretion. Brahmi has adaptogens in it. Adaptogens are compounds present in plants that have the ability to adapt our body to stress and pump up energy. Make it a routine to add Brahmi leaves to your tea and wait for it to banish your stress.

Tulsi/Holy Basil

It's a sacred plant and worshiped all over India even today, it's a mandate to grow tulsi in every Indian house for several health benefits, it's known to reduce stress, blood sugar, and good for heart. Eat 10-12 raw leaves every morning, you can add some fresh leaves to your cup.

Jatamasi/Spikenard

Jatamasi is known for preventing cell damage by antioxidants in it. It's an anti-fatigue, anti- stress herb. The root has therapeutic effects on your brain. It acts as a brain tonic and helps to remove toxins and improve memory and brain functions. Take 1 tbsp. of jatamasi powder and mix with half tsp of hing and add a pinch of lauh basma. This mixture is known for treating melancholic depression.

Ashwagandha/Indian Ginseng

This miracle herb is known to reduce stress and anxiety, lowers the levels of cholesterol and triglycerides. In men, it increases testosterone levels and promotes fertility, helps fight depression, and improves brain function. Add ashwagandha root into boiling water and boil for 15 minutes and add lemon and honey to it.

Ayurvedic Must-Have Spices in Your Kitchen

Cumin is popular among Indian and Mexican cuisines. It is known for balancing all three doshas. Add dry roasted or ground cumin on fresh yogurt, or make a refreshing lassi, blend yogurt, add a pinch of salt and half tsp cumin powder, water (50-50). Make a salad dressing by combining this cumin powder with minced ginger, lemon juice, salt, and black pepper to steamed carrots or cooked white beans, or simply sauté cumin seeds in ghee, and add this to legumes or lentil soups.

Cinnamon

We all love cinnamon rolls, but did you know cinnamon promotes our health by unclogging the respiratory passages, making breathing easy and promotes healthy Joints and bones. Add some cinnamon into your smoothies, milkshakes or rice puddings. Drink some warm milk with cinnamon before going to bed.

Mustard Seeds

Although mustard seeds have gained popularity lately as microgreens, usage of mustard seeds and oil is very common since ancient India. Mustard oil can be helpful in people with elevated lipid levels, diabetes, cardiac issues, skin diseases and neurological disorders. Add mustard seeds to hot ghee or mustard oil and sauté them and use it as salad dressing.

Boswellia

Indian frankincense is a spice with anti-inflammatory properties. It helps in reducing joint pain and increase range of movement and mobility in people with rheumatoid and osteoarthritis, enhances oral health and fight oral infections. In Crohn's disease and ulcerative colitis, it improves digestion, as well as increase lung's capacity for breathing in people with chronic asthma. It also fights against leukemia and breast cancer. One can take 300- 500 mg orally two to three times in a day according to general dosage guidelines.

Asafoetida/Hing

For western cuisines, the usage of asafoetida dates back to centuries during the Roman Empire. But for Indians, they have been adding it in every curry they make on daily basis. Indians add it to the food to prevent digestive problems. Hing has a phyto-chemical known as ferulic acid which is anti-cancerous, anti-inflammatory, antineoplastic, anti-tumor, anti-mutagenic, anti-spasmodic, hepato-protective, antiviral, anti-bacterial, and antioxidant properties. Looks like we have every "anti" word from a medical dictionary!

Basic Equipment in an Ayurvedic Kitchen

"Food as Medicine" is the mantra of Ayurveda. To prepare the food, which also benefits you as a medicine, one must setup a proper kitchen environment. To do that, you'll be needing several appliances, tools, and cookware items.

Don't you worry about that. It's not rocket science. Here, I'm go going to tell you what kind of equipment you need for a Ayurvedic kitchen. You can get most of them at your local store. If not, you can always order them online and get them at your doorstep in a matter of days.

Ayurvedic Cookware

The basic tools in your kitchen are none other than the cookware. Whether it is a pot, pan, or a plate, cookware is the basic requirement for any kitchen, let alone an Ayurvedic kitchen.

So, here are a few items you must have:

Two to four pots, along with lids. If your needs are moderate, get two-quart and four-quart pots.

One frying pan or a sauté pan with a lid.

One pressure cooker. To be honest, I can't really help you here on choosing the size. It would be best for you to choose it yourself, considering the number of people in your family.

A paring knife and a chef's knife. Getting a couple of quality knives is a no-brainer. Make sure that you investigate the quality of it, before buying from the store. If you're going online, check out the reviews.

Electric pressure cooker. Also known as "Instant Pot," this appliance helps you to warm, sauté, cook rice, soups, and beans. They come with timers, which helps you schedule cooking. You can even leave the house, relaxed, since the cooker does the work according to the pre-set timer.

One strainer. Make sure that you get one with a high-quality mesh.

A couple of mixing bowls.

Cooking utensils such as vegetable peeler, serving spoons, wooden and stainless steel spoons.

Cutting board, preferably wooden.

Rolling pan to make chapatis/tortillas.

Some Helpful Tips to Follow While Choosing Cooking Vessels

Steel, non-stick, and glass cookware are pretty common in modern-day kitchens. However, Ayurveda has something else to offer. As I've said earlier, Ayurveda is a complete medical system that only focuses on food, but also several other aspects related to it.

Ayurveda dictates high importance on different types of cookware for cooking different types of food. It simply means that you have to cook a food item with a particular cookware for better benefits. Anyhow, let's talk about the different cookware materials and the foods that should be cooked with them.

Copper: If you're cooking rice, Copper is the best metal. Use the cookware that's made with copper to reap the full benefits. Moreover, not only for cooking, but it's also very beneficial to store water overnight. You can start your day by drinking the water stored in a copper vessel and enjoy all the benefits of this metal.

Copper boosts collagen, making it very good for your skin. If you're a Kapha, say no more, and start using copper vessels in your kitchen. As it helps in dealing with excessive weight gain, congestion, and coughs, you shouldn't neglect having copper vessels. It also helps in detoxifying your body, enhances the hemoglobin levels, helps in better secretion of bile, and many more.

Bronze: Unfortunately, not a lot of people are using vessels or cookware made out of this metal. But, little do the people know the amazing benefits of this metal. If you're vata, bronze is a natural pacifier for you.

It helps in managing several health conditions such as irritability, nervous mood swings, dry skin, and many more. Moreover, people with obesity, poor eyesight, and skin issues could be greatly benefited. But, remember one thing, never use ghee in a vessel made out of bronze.

Brass: If you're looking to strengthen your immunity, immediately start using brass vessels to store your drinking water. This metal also benefits people who're suffering from aggressions, burning sensations, low hemoglobin count, and several skin conditions. And hey, brass vessels also eliminate germs from the water stored in it, in as low as 4 hours.

Clay: I can't stress this enough, Clay pots are the best cookware to prepare your food. It's almost shocking that whatever you cook, using a clay vessel or pot greatly enhances the taste of it. Moreover, not only the taste, but it also provides a lot of health benefits too.

Ayurveda highly encourages cooking using a clay pot. Clay comes with good insulator and porosity properties, making it a better choice than almost all other cooking utensil materials. Clay pots enable high levels of moisture and heat circulation evenly throughout the vessel or pot. This highly enhances the quality and taste of your food. Moreover, this factor also helps in lowering the levels of nutrient and moisture loss from your food.

Iron: Pretty much every grandmother of this generation used to cook in ironware kitchen utensils, back in their day. Cast iron vessels greatly reduce the need for oil, which makes it very good for people having cardiovascular issues.

Additionally, you can say goodbye to your iron deficiency issues, by using cast iron cookware. But, keep in mind, that ironware utensils require seasoning, where you'd need to add a coating of heating and oil.

Ayurvedic Pantry Staples

Ayurvedic dishes require a lot of legumes, grains, and other staples. They add taste, flavor, and several health benefits to the food.

Here are a few Ayurvedic pantry staples you need to add to your grocery shopping list:

Whole and split mungs: Mung beans are highly nutritive and easily digestible legumes. Split mungs are better for quick cooking.

Brown and white rice: There are several types of rice available. Among them, brown and white rice is the most commonly used.

Adzuki beans: These beans need 6-8 hours of soaking before they're cooked.

Barley: If you ever get bored with rice, you can replace it with barley. Highly nutritive and good for your digestive system.

Ayurvedic spices: You can't cook an Ayurvedic dish without using spices. I guess you got the point. You can't afford to neglect buying spices when you're shopping for groceries.

Mineral salt: A highly important staple used in almost all Ayurvedic dishes, mineral salt is an integral part of an Ayurvedic kitchen.

Cooking as a Path to Awakening

For many, cooking is just a chore or a task, waiting to be completed. However, for me, it has been a therapeutic experience. To be precise, anything you do, if you're focused on that one single thing, at that moment, it's a therapy. And when it comes to cooking, it's all more important, as it's related to the food we eat.

Over the last few years, I've developed a strong skill of maintaining a conscious relationship with my food. First, I sit a pray for a couple of minutes every time I'm about to cook or eat. I simply thank the universe for providing the food. Then, whenever I cook or eat, I focus solely on that. No watching TikTok or scrolling through my Facebook feed. It has helped me enjoy the process even more.

Oh, one more thing. Cooking has also benefited me as a self-care therapy. Yep, it's a form of self-care, since you take care of yourself by cooking the food you enjoy. Also, as it's a repetitive process, your brain becomes accustomed to the process of focusing on something, and accomplishing it every day. I'd say, it's even a form of meditation too.

Ayurvedic Recipes to Treat Anxiety and Depression

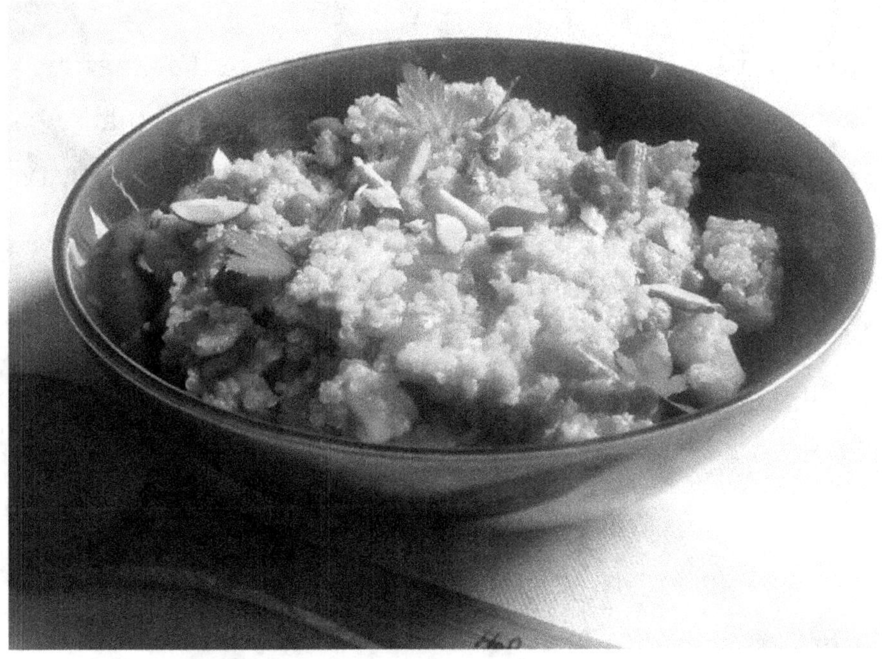

As I've said earlier, Ayurveda says that "You are what you eat." Actually, this is the core principle of this medical system. And, if you think about it, it really makes sense. I mean, if you eat junk food every day, your health becomes junk too, doesn't it?

So, it's safe to say that if you eat healthily, your body stays healthy, too! Look, we all know and feel the temptation to eat tasty junk food every now and then. If it stays every now and then, it's okay! However, if you increase the frequency of unhealthy dietary habits, then it becomes a problem worth worrying about.

Anyhow, here, I would like to give you some of the amazing Ayurvedic recipes I've personally tried and used. Actually, even to this day, I use these recipes and cook awesome, tasty, and healthy food day in and day out. I've also focused on providing recipes that are suitable for almost everyone, every dosha, and every season. So, without wasting any time, let's get into the recipes.

Ayurvedic Teas

Who doesn't like to sip a tea, while reading your daily news brief, watching a cool Netflix show, or simply relaxing in your backyard?!

The land where Ayurveda originated from, India, is also infamous for its tea collection. Here are a few Ayurvedic tea recipes:

CCF Digest Tea

CCF stands for coriander, cumin, and fennel. This tea is ideal for all doshas. Cumin works great for vata, while coriander suits pitta, especially in improving the digestive system. Finally, fennel is a key ingredient that helps all doshas including kapha. Moreover, CCF tea is good for all seasons. So, if you like it very much, you can sip it all day, all year. Other than its digestive benefits, it also detoxifies.

Ingredients:

Cumin seeds: ¼ teaspoon

Coriander seeds: ¼ teaspoon

Fennel seeds: ¼ teaspoon

Water: 6 cups

Preparation

1. Take all the ingredients and place them in a big pot. After boiling them, bring down the heat to low, cover the pot, and

let it simmer for 10 minutes.

2. Now, it's time to strain it and remove the seeds. Finally, keep the tea in a thermos. You can now have the tea ready. Sip it whenever you want throughout the day.

Ginger, Honey, and Lemon Tea

With a multitude of tastes, this tea is delicious, since it's sweet, pungent, sour, and warm. Not only it's medicinal, it's comforting too. Moreover, this tea helps you strengthen your immune system. Make sure that take it often, especially in Spring and Winter. If you're suffering from cold, this is the go-to tea.

Ingredients

Fresh Ginger: 1 piece

Water: 4 cups

Lemon juice of 1 lemon

Raw Honey: 2 tablespoons

<u>Preparation</u>

1. Chop the ginger after peeling it. Take a pot, fill it with water, and place the ginger in it. Then, cover the pot and let the content boil. Now, reduce the heat and let it simmer for about 10 minutes. Now, switch off the heat and steep it for 5 more minutes.

2. Then, wait for the tea to cool down, so that you can remove the ginger chips.

3. Now, you can stir the tea with a tablespoon of raw honey and enjoy sipping the delicious tea.

Rose Fennel Tea

A rose is a personification of calm, cool, and soothing. Imagine how good it would be, if you can have a tea with it. Fennel is a sweet and calming digestive ingredient. Add to them, mint, which is a refreshing element. When you combine all these three ingredients, you get a tasty tea which suits Summer the best.

<u>Ingredients</u>

Water: 2 cups

Fennels seeds: 1 teaspoon

Mint leaves: 5 leaves

Rose water: 2 tablespoons

Preparation

1. Take a saucepan, and use it to boil the water.

2. Put those fennel seeds in it and let it bowl, with heat set to low.

3. Wait for 3 minutes so that the mixture is simmered enough. Now, switch off the heat. Wait for 5 more minutes, so that the seeds are steeped.

4. Add the mint leaves and rose water and stir. Now, you have completed making delicious rose fennel tea.

Ayurvedic Tonics

Ayurvedic tonics are a bunch of post-lunch drinks that help you digest the food better, calm your belly down, and ultimately provide a cooling effect. Not only, they're tasty to drink, they're also highly beneficial to your stomach. Moreover, they also offer other benefits such as improving your immune system, balancing your dosha, providing vital nutrients, and many more. Here are a few Ayurvedic tonics you must make and consume often.

Digestive Lassi

India is not only famous for its tea collection, but also for its wide range of lassis as well. Almost everyone completes their meal with a lassi. After a heavy meal, your stomach definitely appreciates a cooling tonic, which is why we're now about to learn digestive lassi. This lassi is especially beneficial and relieving, when you're suffering from diarrhea.

Ingredients

Yogurt: 1 cup

Raw honey: 1 teaspoon

Vanilla extract: 1 teaspoon

Cinnamon: A pinch

Freshly grated nutmeg: A pinch

Cloves: A pinch

Pink salt: A pinch

Black pepper: A pinch

Water: 1 cup

Preparation

1. Use a blender to blend all the above-mentioned ingredients.

2. Enjoy the delicious lassi after having your meal.

Cucumber Mint Cooler

The name gives it away; this is an amazing cooler, especially in the Summer. It comes with tons of electrolytes, which not only cools you down but also acts as an instant energy-booster. If you're a pitta, you must definitely include this in your daily food menu. But hey, it works well for other doshas too.

Ingredients

Persian cucumber: One chopped into a few pieces

Lime juice of one lime

Mint leaves: 6

Pink salt: A pinch

Water: 1 cup

Preparation

1. Take all the ingredients and blend them with a blender. Do this until all the items are pureed properly.

2. Now, pour it into the glass and garnish the cooler with a

couple of additional mint leaves.

Golden Milk

This is one of the best Ayurvedic tonics suitable for all doshas. Since it contains turmeric, which helps in cleansing blood, the lymphatic system, and other body systems, it is highly beneficial to your health. It also improves blood circulation, dissolves blood clots and tumors, promotes ideal menstruation, and heals soft tissue injuries. This tonic also has coconut milk.

Ingredients

Whole milk: 2 cups

Ground turmeric: 1 tablespoon

Black pepper: A pinch

Cardamom: A pinch

Preparation

1. Place all the above-mentioned ingredients on a saucepan. Whisk it gently and turn the heat to low. Wait for a 3-4 minutes.

2. Now, serve the tonic and drink it while it's warm.

Ayurvedic Breakfasts

What's better than starting your day with a tasty breakfast? Well, there's something better that that. Yep, it is when your tasty breakfast is also a healthy one. No, I'm not asking you to consider eating raw leaves and veggies for your breakfast. However, I'm trying to say that a healthy breakfast can be tasty too. In Ayurveda, there's room for a lot of flexibility. So, don't worry and think that you have to sacrifice taste if you're planning on eating a healthy food. Anyhow, here are a few thoughtfully curated Ayurvedic breakfast recipes for you.

Buckwheat Pancakes

Who doesn't love pancakes?! I mean, it's one of the most commonly eaten breakfasts around the world. However, here's the twist. With the help of Ayurveda, you can have your pancakes not only tasty, but also super-healthy too. Cardamom is a very good spice, however, for a better taste, you can replace it with cinnamon.

Ingredients

Buckwheat flour: 2 cups

Baking powder: 1 teaspoon

Ground cardamom: ½ teaspoon

A pinch of pink salt

Eggs: 1

Milk: 3½ cups

Lime zest: 1 teaspoon

Ghee: 1 teaspoon

Maple syrup: as desired to taste and garnish, but not too much!

Preparation

1. Preheat your oven and set it to the lowest keep warm setting.

2. Take a large bowl and mix baking powder, salt, and cinnamon with the buckwheat flour.

3. Stir and whisk the egg.

4. Pour the milk into the mixture and stir it constantly.

5. Now, melt the ghee in a frying pan. As it gets heated, cover the bottom of the pan with batter. Now, follow the usual pancake-cooking steps, keeping pancakes warm in the oven until you're ready to serve them.

6. Finally, when the pancakes are done, serve them with maple syrup.

Rice Pudding

Grains are some of the most-used staples of Ayurveda. Add in some spices, you will have a tasty and healthy breakfast. Rice pudding is a basic yet effective Ayurvedic breakfast item, as it not only offers a delicious taste, but also is very easy to cook. Moreover, it also offers tons of energy, which is more than enough to start your day.

Ingredients

Basmati rice: 1 cup

Ghee: 1 tablespoon

Ground cardamom: ¼ tablespoon

Pinch salt

Boiling water: 1 cup

Almond milk: 1 cup

Dates: 4

Golden raisins: ½ cup

Preparation

1. Rinse and clean the rice for a couple of minutes.

2. Take a saucepan, set it to medium heat, and melt the ghee. Then, add in the Ground cardamom and wait for one minute.

3. Stir the salt and rice, so that the grains are coated properly.

4. Now, slowly, add the water.

5. Finally, pour the almond milk, set the heat to medium, and wait for 20 minutes before you add in raising and dates. Now, set the heat to low and wait for 10 more minutes. That's it! You now have your Ayurvedic rice pudding.

Amarnath Chai Porridge

Here's your dose of exotic Ayurvedic breakfast. As it is full of spices, it eliminates the toxics from your body, improves your agni, and fire you up for an energetic day. This breakfast is my favorite, as it somehow brightens up my mood, especially whenever I wake up all gloomy and doomy.

<u>Ingredients</u>

Ghee: 1 teaspoon

Autumn spice blend: 1 teaspoon

Ground cloves: ½ tablespoon

Salt

Amarnath: 1 cup

Almond milk: 2 cups

Apples: 1

Flaxseed: 1 teaspoon

Preparation

1. Take a pot, heat it on medium setting and then melt the ghee.

2. After that, stir in the cloves, salt, and spice blend.

3. Then, pour the almond milk, apple pieces, amaranth, flaxseed, and let it boil.

4. The final step is to simmer it for 20 minutes on low heat settings.

Brahmi Pesto

Did you know this antidepressant herb can not only give you mental clarity but can also make a tasty pesto. I love this recipe, because it's easy to make, tasty to eat, and ultimately comes with a lot of health benefits. Moreover, brahmi pesto goes well with a lot of dishes.

Ingredients

Olive oil: ½ cup

Black pepper powder: ½ teaspoon

Fresh grated ginger: ½ teaspoon

Rock salt: ½ teaspoon

Pecans: ½ teaspoon

Fennel powder: ¼ teaspoon

Fresh basil: ½ cup

Coriander powder: ½ teaspoon

Chopped kale: 3 cups

1 mashed avocado

Brahmi powder: ¼ cup

Lime juice: 1 tablespoon

Preparation

1. Heat the pan and add some olive oil. Once it's warm, add the grated fresh ginger, salt, black pepper, and pecans.

2. Now simmer the flame until the aroma lasts, and add coriander, fennel powders, and basil.

3. Simmer for a minute; lastly add in the brahmi and kale. Now splash some water and cover the pan until kale is soft. Turn off the heat and let it cool. Add them to a blender and blend it along with avocado, olive oil, and lime juice. Serve it

as salad dressing, or spread this sauce on pearl barley, pasta, rice.

Ayurvedic Lunches

I'd say, lunch is the most important meal of the day. I know, many people would consider breakfast as the most significant, but I differ with that, and I have my own reasons. Anyhow, lunch is what gets you moving until the night, where you get off your duty. Also, lunch is where you eat the most. So, it's very important to make sure that you have your lunch, not only tasty, but also healthy. Over the last few years, I've been exclusively eating Ayurvedic food items for my lunch. Oh yeah, they're so good that I've almost forgotten how the usual lunch meals taste like. So, here are a few of my favorite Ayurvedic lunch recipes.

Spinach Paneer

Thanks to the age-old classic cartoon, "Popeye," Spinach has become an important part of our lives. It not only offers rich amounts of iron, but also provides you many vital nutrients as well. Paneer comes with its unique set of benefits. Combined together, we get the spinach paneer, which is very easy to make, and also goes light on your stomach.

Ingredients

Milk: 2 cups

Lemons: 1

Ghee: 1 teaspoon

Seasonal spice blend: 1 teaspoon

Nutmeg: ¼ teaspoon

Chopped spinach: 4 cups

Coconut milk: ½ cup

Preparation

1. Boil the milk moderately, and then squeeze half of lemon into it.

2. Turn off the heat and let it cool down for a few minutes.

3. Take a strainer, and pour the milk through it. This step

removes all the unnecessary liquid, and only the mixture remains.

4. Now, flatten the paneer, with the help of a cheesecloth and a plate.

5. It's time to melt the ghee on medium heat setting. Add the nutmeg and spice blend to it.

6. Now cook it for 3 minutes by adding the spinach. Also, pour the coconut milk, lower down the heat settings to low.

7. Crumble the paneer and add it to the spinach mixture. Wait for one minute before switching off the heat.

8. Sprinkle the remaining half of lemon juice and serve it warm.

Spring Pea Salad

Crunchy peas are not only tasty to eat, they're also very healthy for your gut, as they're very good for your digestive system. Add to them some veggies, spices, and lemon juice, you get a very tasty and healthy salad. It's suitable for people, seasons, and doshas. Moreover, it just takes 5 minutes of your time to prepare it.

Ingredients

Mayonnaise: 1 tablespoon

Dijon mustard: 1 teaspoon

Minced ginger: 1 teaspoon

Lemon juice: 1 tablespoon

Salt

Black pepper

Snap peas: 2 cups

Shredded cabbage: 1 cup

Sliced radish: 1 cup

Chopped watercress: 1 cup

Preparation

1. Take a small bowl, mix the ingredients such as mustard, mayonnaise, lemon juice, and ginger. Then, season it with pepper and salt.

2. Take the cabbage, watercress, radish, and peas. Now, add the dressing and toss it well.

Kitchari

If you're looking for a light, easy-to-digest, tasty, and refreshing meal, Kitchari is the way to go. This dish is extremely easy to prepare, highly beneficial to your health, and most importantly very tasty. You can make it in about half an hour and serve it to yourself and your loved ones whenever you feel like having a good lunch.

Ingredients

Basmati rice: 1 cup

Beans: 1 cup

Ghee: 1 tablespoon

Spice blend: 1 teaspoon

Basic broth: 5 cups

Kombu: 1 piece

Shredded coconut: ¼ cup

Chopped vegetables: 1 cup

Black pepper

Fresh mint

Olive oil

Preparation

1. Use cool water to rinse the beans and rice. Then, set them aside to drain.

2. Take a large pot, use medium-heat settings, to melt the

ghee. Then, add the spice blend slowly.

3. Now, place the rice and beans in the spicy ghee mixture.

4. It's time to add the kombu and coconut and then change the heat settings to low.

5. Let it cook for 20 minutes before adding the vegetables. Let it cook for 10 more minutes.

6. Season the mixture with pepper and salt. Finally, add the fresh mint and olive oil.

Ayurvedic Dinners

Let's talk about the dinner. You're done with your work, arrived home, tired, and hungry. What would you like? A tasty meal? Or a healthy meal? I'd say, why not both? Gone are the days of sacrificing taste for health. With Ayurveda, you can now go to bed, having eaten a stupendously tasty food, that also offers a plethora of health benefits. Moreover, it's important that you eat healthy food before going bed, if you're suffering from any of the mental health issues such as anxiety.

Restorative Shoots & Roots Broth

I bet you probably have never tasted something like this dish. This is a unique type of dish, that includes a root and shoot. Are you confused? Well, I'm talking about roots like a carrot, and shoots like a celery. Not only they're rich in several nutrients and vitamins, but also offer several benefits to patients with mental health problems. On top of that, they also provide heaps of energy for you to last a good night's sleep.

Ingredients

Beet: 1

Daikon radish: 1

Celery stalk: 1

Water: 4 cups

Salt

Black pepper

<u>**Preparation**</u>

1. Chop the shoots and roots, celery, beet, and radish.

2. Using a soup pot, place the chopper vegetables, and add salt, pepper, and water to it.

3. After letting it boil for a few minutes, turn down the heat setting to low, and simmer it for 15 more minutes.

4. That's it, you're done preparing this tasty and easily-digestible Ayurvedic dinner.

Ginger Broccolini

Cancer hates Broccoli. Actually, it hates the entire cabbage spectrum, under which broccoli falls. Anyhow, ginger broccolini is an excellent dinner dish, which goes easy on your stomach, provides all the necessary vitamins before going to bed. The taste is amazing too, with bitter and astringent blend, it's very delicious, I'd say.

<u>**Ingredients**</u>

Broccolini: 1 bunch

Ghee: 1 tablespoon

Minced ginger: 1 tablespoon

Lemon zest: 1 teaspoon

Lemon juice: 1 tablespoon

Black pepper

Salt

Preparation

1. Boil the salted water in a large pot.

2. Take a large bowl and fill it with ice and water.

3. Immerse the broccolini and drain it in the ice water.

4. Now, take a skillet and use it to melt ghee under medium heat settings.

5. Add zest and ginger to it.

6. Now, take out the broccolini, drain it, and place it in the skillet. Let it cook for a couple of minutes.

7. Then, drizzle the lemon juice onto it, season it with pepper and salt.

Curried Green Beans

Curry is a vaguely used term. I'll tell you what it's about. A curry is a food dish, primarily made of spices. Usually, we add in some vegetables, to make different types of curries. I'd say, it's one of the tastiest food items, especially, since it's from Ayurveda, we get immense number of health benefits too.

<u>Ingredients</u>

Salt: 1 teaspoon

Chopped green beans: 1 pound

Ghee: 2 tablespoons

Brown mustard seed: ½ teaspoon

Minced ginger: 1 teaspoon

Spice blend: ½ teaspoon

Chopped hazelnuts: ½ cup

Tamari: 1 teaspoon

Black pepper

Flat-leaf parsley

Preparation

1. Take a pot of water and boil it. Then, add a teaspoon of salt.

2. Take a bowl and fill it with ice and water.

3. Now, add the beans to the hot water and let if cook for a couple of minutes.

4. After that, drain the beans, and place them in the cold water,

5. After sometime, take out the beans, and let them dry.

6. Get a saucepan, heat it on medium settings, and use it to melt 1 tablespoon of ghee.

7. Place the mustard seeds, and immediately stir in spice blend and ginger as soon as the seeds being to pop.

8. Now, let it cook for a minute.

9. Take out the beans, and pour them in the spicy blend of ghee. Cook it for five minutes.

10. Then, take another pan, melt another tablespoon of ghee, and add the hazelnuts.

11. Finally, add the tamari to the beans, season it with pepper, salt, and hazelnuts. Don't forget to top it off with leaf parsley.

Ayurvedic Snacks and Sweets

You don't have to ring in your favorite junk food supplier, to munch on some tasty snacks, while working from your home. Yep, Ayurveda comes to your rescue, here as well. Ayurveda has solutions for pretty much everything related to food. And, on contrary with the popular snacks, Ayurvedic snacks aren't just for tasty bites, but also healthy bites too.

Flatbread Pizza

Gone are the days of worrying too much about eating a pizza. You can have a pizza, and stay healthy too. Oh, I'm not talking about your regular pizza here. Rather, I'm discussing Pizza with an Ayurvedic twist. Oh, I can see you're salivating already! Let's not waste any time, here's the recipe.

Ingredients

Ghee: 1 teaspoon

Spice blend: 1 teaspoon

Zucchini: 1

Chapatis/tortillas: 2

Basil pesto: ½ cup

Paneer: ½ cup

<u>Preparation</u>

1. Preheat your over to precisely 350°F.

2. Take a saucepan and use it to melt the ghee. Make sure you do it under medium heat settings.

3. Pour in the spice blend, and gently move the pan for it to mix. Now, add the zucchini.

4. Take a slotted spoon, and use it to move the zucchini onto a plate.

5. Then, take the chapatis/tortillas and pour the ghee and zucchini onto them.

6. Add a layer of pesto on the chapatis. Take the paneer, and crumble them to spread it across the zucchini evenly.

7. Bake the chapatis for about 10 minutes. After it's done, wait for a couple of minutes to let it cool down, before serving it.

Cauli Tacos

I don't know about you, but for me, Tacos is the favorite snack to munch on. I don't care what time of the day it is, I can eat this snack all day, every day. And, it gets even better, when it's Ayurvedic, since I can enjoy vast health benefits too, while biting on my favorite snack item. And the best thing is, 10 minutes is all it takes to cook this dish.

Ingredients

Ghee: 3 tablespoons

Chopped cauliflower pieces

Salt

Black pepper

Paprika: ½ teaspoon

Mayonnaise: ¼ cup

Lime juice: ½

Pickle juice: 1 tablespoon

Chapatis/tortillas: 4

Avocado mash

Preparation

1. Use a large skillet to melt the ghee. After it's reasonably hot, take the cauliflower pieces and add them.

2. Cook it for approximately 8 minutes, while stirring it now and then.

3. Take a slotted spoon, use to take out the cauliflower pieces and move them onto a plate.

4. Season them with paprika, pepper, and salt.

5. Take a small bowl, and mix the lime juice and mayonnaise

in it.

6. Now, finally, assemble the tacos. Take the chapatti, put some cauliflower pieces at the center of it, and add some white sauce and avocado mash.

Nutty Apple Pie

Oh no, I'm not going to do the mistake of excluding an Ayurvedic sweet recipe. More than that, I'd hate myself if I miss a pie recipe. Oh yeah, the ever-green sizzling and sweetish dish, that we all savor with joy. A pie is one of the only food items that's suitable for all occasions, weathers, and times. So, here it is, the Ayurvedic nutty apple pie recipe.

<u>Ingredients for the Piecrust</u>

Pecans: 2 cups

Medjool dates: 10

Ghee: 1 tablespoon

Ground cinnamon

Nutmeg

Salt

Ingredients for the Pie Filling

Lemon Juice: 2 tablespoons

Maple syrup: 1 tablespoon

Vanilla extract: 1 teaspoon

Melted ghee: 1 teaspoon

Spice blend: ½ teaspoon

Sliced Red Delicious or other red apples: 4-6

Raw honey

Preparing the Pie Crust

1. Preheat your oven accurately to 350°F.

2. Use a flying pan to toast the pecans. Use medium heat settings, while also stirring them in ghee.

3. Now, use a blender to mix the nutmeg, dates, salt, and cinnamon.

4. After that, place the pecans in the blender and blend them for a minute.

5. Once it's done, take the mixture out and move it onto a pie pan of precisely 9-inch. Spread the crust evenly.

6. Bake it for approximately 5 minutes.

Preparing the Pie Filling

1. Take a large bowl and use it to whisk together ghee, vanilla extract, lemon juice, spices, and maple syrup.

2. Now, combine it with apple slices and toss it gently.

3. Start with one apple piece, place it at the center of piecrust, and make a rose petal pattern with the rest of pieces.

4. Cover the entire pie with the apple slices. Once it's done, sprinkle the juice over it.

5. Use foil to cover the pie and bake it for up to half an hour.

6. Then, remove the foil and wait for 5 minutes for it to cool down a bit.

7. Take the raw honey and drizzle the pie with it.

Final Words

Now, finally, we've arrived to the last part of this book. Honestly, I enjoyed quite a lot writing this. And, I hope that you've also enjoyed reading it. If you've found any mistakes, or errors, please forgive me. Writing is not my forte, but I've tried my best putting all the information together.

Whatever I've written, it was honest, fact-based, and also based on my personal experiences. Oh, I've considered several reputed researches too. Moreover, I'm primarily a dental assistant, who miraculously found passion in Ayurveda, and the lifestyle based on this amazing and ancient health system.

I want to wrap this book up with a few tips that could help you in the long run. These health and lifestyle tips, based on Ayurveda, changed my life. Most importantly, they helped me overcome my anxiety and depression that I've developed over the period of my horrible, painful, and depressing PCOS days. I so hope that these tips also help you with whatever you're having trouble with. Moreover, I'm writing these tips, not only for your physical wellbeing, but also your mental wellbeing.

I make sure that I include all these tips in such a way that is helpful for you in developing a strong and healthy discipline. Remember, discipline is very important while fighting the evil of mental health issues. And, discipline also helps you develop a strong will, which helps you in combating your depression and anxiety. Finally, before going to these tips, I would like to ask you one thing. If you like this book, and the information in it, please be kind and give it a positive review on whatever platform you happen to find it.

You see, my friend, health is not just physical. Actually, from my experience, it's more mental. Or, should I say, that they are both inter-linked, and if one gets sick, the other would also follow the same path? Yes, if your mind gets sick, your body does too, and vice versa. So, it's important that you take care of both. Especially, when you're battling any mental health condition, you not only should focus on your mental wellbeing, but also your physical wellbeing too.

I've been a strict follower of these below Ayurvedic tips, and honestly, I've never felt better. Now, every day is blissful for me. And, I honestly want you to feel the same, waking up with an awesome mind-set, and conquering your day like a Viking. But, please, keep this in mind; it's always a long journey, no shortcuts here. So, follow these tips consistently for at least two months, before expecting significant results.

Defeat the sun at who-wakes-up-first challenge. Yes, it's very important to get up early in morning. Oh no, by early, I don't mean 7 or 8 in the morning. You should try and get up before the sun even starts shining. Or, for simplicity, I'd say 5:00 in the morning is a good time.

Start your day with a fat pizza. Alright, I'm kidding, please don't do that. A healthy way to start your day is with a prayer. You can pray to whomever your like, in whatever way you prefer. For me, I really like to pray to the universe just to say thank you and express my never-ending gratitude for all the good in not only my life, but for the good everywhere.

After that, drink a glass of water that's not too hot or too cold. Ideally, take a copper vessel, and fill it with water the night before. And then, when you wake up in the morning, have the water. It helps your digestive system, and your excretive system as well.

Ayurvedic system suggests you to squat, rather than sit while you evacuate the bodily wastes. Even several modern day studies show that squatting is far better than sitting. If you're having troubles with bowel movements, you must definitely try this tip. Do it for a few days, as it takes some time for your body to get used to the new way.

It's very important to clean your sensory organs like your eyes, mouth, and tongue. Clean your face using cold water. Also, rinse your mouth with some warm water. It helps you get rid of the bacteria that's on the surface layers of your tongue and teeth. Also, with cold water, clean your eyes. After that, gently massage your eyelids. For better eye care, you can also try blinking your eyes for about 5-7 times. Finally, once you're done with cleaning these parts, take a clean towel and dry your face.

You know, digestion is one of the most important bodily functions. However, when I talk about digestion, don't think that I'm just talking about abdomen alone. Tongue is very important for a better digestion. Because, saliva is produced over the tongue, it plays a very key role in the digestion of food. For a better and healthy tongue, scrape your tongue, as it helps you eliminate all types of bacteria, presiding over it.

How can I overlook the importance of clean teeth? Well, I don't. Bad and unhealthy teeth can affect your overall wellbeing very negatively. Because, after all, you chew your food with them. You can use a high-quality tooth brush and a toothpaste. However, if you're interested in the Ayurvedic way, clean your teeth with a neem stick. It possesses high amounts of detoxifying elements, that not only clean your teeth, but other parts of the mouth as well.

Now, would you like to be fit and flexible? Well, fitness not only makes you look good, but it also promotes you to feel good as well. Your confident skyrockets, when your body is in a good shape. When I was dealing with PCOS, I gained a lot of weight, which badly dented my confidence. However, I've worked on myself, following strict yoga regime, which not only helped regain my shape, but it also played a crucial role in getting a positive mind set, attitude, and my confidence back. So, make yoga a daily activity.

Breathing exercises are some of the most underrated wellbeing activities in the world. Especially, the western societies have overlooked it for a long time. Pranayama has been an integral part of the Ayurvedic and yogic culture. These ancient breathing techniques, offer a plethora of benefits like a strong respiratory system, enhanced blood circulatory system, improved endurance, and more importantly promotes a clean mind.

To complete the whole physical and mental wellbeing

regime, I would like you to include meditation as well. When you're suffering from anxiety, depression, PTSD, or any other mental health problem, I can't stress enough on how important it is, to meditate daily. Honestly, daily meditation has been the real game changer for me, as I've struggle when it came to having a clear mind.

Alright, I guess that's pretty much it. Look, I've been following this holistic lifestyle for the last few years, and I'm now living a positive, confident, and a very happy life. I would like you to have a positive and happy life. I hope these tips and information help you achieve that. Finally, before ending this book, I'd like to thank my grandma, who guided me to the path of Ayurveda. And you, thank you so much for reading my book!